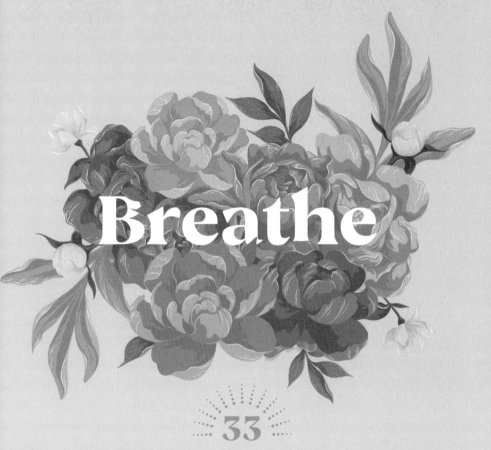

Breathe

33
Simple Breathwork Practices

SHANILA SATTAR

ROCK
POINT

Contents

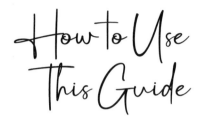

How to Use This Guide

First, let me start off by letting you know that there is absolutely no wrong way to do breathwork.

In this guide, I've outlined thirty-three incredible breathing techniques that are made easy for everyone. And I mean everyone. Many of these techniques are ancient, and some are my own personal creations from practicing breathwork over the years. These easy, accessible, and holistic tools can support well-being and can be life changing, as we're all learning to take better care of ourselves and each other, and enhance the collective experience. I thought long and hard about creating this breathwork guide and how it will benefit you in your real life. I wanted you to have something that you will actually use.

There are going to be practices in this guide that will make you say, "Yes! I love this one! I'm going to keep this one." There will be other exercises in here that you're not going to resonate with as much. That's okay. The goal of having this guide in your hands is so you can pick and choose the exercises and techniques that really resonate with you, work for you, and are what you need in your own life; these will be the ones that you truly enjoy practicing.

I've organized the exercises into a few categories:

MOOD

These are the techniques that will shift your mood. Use these practices
if you're grumpy, feeling low, or not feeling like yourself.
Mood-boosting breathwork practices will help you feel confident,
empowered, centered, and high vibe.

ENERGY

These are the techniques that will uplift and elevate your energy.
Use these practices if you're feeling a lull in energy, focus, inspiration,
or creativity. Energy-boosting breathwork practices will help you
pump feel-good hormones throughout your body, so you'll feel
energized and awakened.

INNER HEALING

These are the techniques that will promote deep inner healing.
Use these practices if you are on a self-healing journey, are working
on energetic alignment, or are doing deep subconscious work.
Inner healing practices tend to be best if you leave time for grounding
and integration after your practice.

RELAXATION AND GROUNDING

These are the techniques that will help you relax and recenter back into your body. Use these techniques if you want to ground your energy, ease tension, reduce stress, or relax your muscles. Relaxation and grounding practices are perfect to do in the middle of your busy days.

SLEEP

These are the techniques that will help you sleep better. Use these techniques when you are ready to go to bed and call it a night. Prepare your nighttime space and do your nightly routine; these practices will help calm your body, ease the chatter in your mind, and help you get deep, restful, quality sleep.

Of course, there is a bit of overlap between the categories; for example, exercises that help you relax can also help you sleep and vice versa. When you turn to the guide, **meditate on your intention of what you want to feel after you do a practice**. If you're feeling low energy and want to bring more energy into your body, you'll turn to the energy section of this guide and use a technique in that section.

The techniques outlined in this book are generally safe to practice on an everyday basis. If you have a known medical condition, suffer from any respiratory ailments, have a history of vertigo, or are on any medications that may prevent you from doing prolonged breathing, please consult a medical professional first. Techniques that include holding your breath should not be practiced by anyone who is pregnant or has a history of fainting.

As with any healthy habit, it takes twenty-one to thirty-three days to build a practice. Consistency helps program the subconscious mind and the energetic body to stick with a practice that's going to be incredibly life changing in the long run. That's why I have thirty-three practices in this guide for you: one for each day.

For the first seven days that you use this guide, I invite you to follow along with me daily for seven minutes with your exclusive access to videos of a handful of the breathwork practices in this book (see the link below). You can watch me demonstrate the exercises, practice together, and build your daily practice.

Afterward, you can build your breathwork tool kit, a collection of three to five of the practices that really resonate with you and that you can come back to whenever you want.

Before each practice, you are invited to do a quick check-in about your current state using The Breathwork Inventory (see page 42). **After your practice**, you'll do an easy self-reflection either in a journal or mentally.

Each breathwork technique can be practiced for a few seconds all the way up to several hours. The recommended duration for each practice is a simple seven minutes a day. I encourage you to practice long durations with a certified breathwork facilitator and trained guide.

Any page with this symbol means you can follow along with me at www.alwaysplay.org/breathe.

I've also included a symbol for the exercises that are safe and encouraged for kids. These particular exercises can be really fun to practice with your kids, or for kids to practice on their own.

Introduction

Hello, I'm Shanila, your breathwork guide. I'm a breathwork teacher, a fourth-generation sound healer, creator of the FLOW Breathwork method, women's researcher, and the founder of AlwaysPlay Studios and The Integrative Healing Academy, where I train breathwork facilitators and sound healers and mentor aspiring healers. I've created the world's first healing arts practitioner training program, and my virtual studio thrives on supporting the healing arts, training practitioners, and bringing holistic wellness tools to people all across the world, especially in underserved, underrepresented, and marginalized communities. We've been able to implement a lot of cool programs in women's shelters and youth groups with the support of state grants and community outreach. I also host a fun show called *The Playground Podcast*, which is all about spiritual exploration, self-healing, personal development, and intuitive entrepreneurship.

Through the years, I've had the absolute pleasure of supporting hundreds of practitioners to learn the number one somatic healing tool in the world—breathwork—for life-changing experiences in their communities. Therapists, coaches, doctors, nurses, healers, and guides have been able to use the healing art of breathwork and make an impact in communities that deal with trauma, anxiety, insomnia, addiction, generational healing, collective healing, and so much more.

My background is in research science, technology, and psychology. Coming from a world of linear, logical, and systematic ways of thinking and being, I haven't always been very in tune with my body. As my family moved to the US from Bangladesh, a lot of the healing tools passed down in our family did not translate to my experiences in US society. So, even as someone who is generally healthy,

I found myself experiencing illnesses manifesting in my body out of nowhere. My hair was falling out. I was having panic attacks, insomnia, random bouts of fainting, seasonal depression, and a whole slew of illnesses. All this stemmed from the fact that nobody really taught me the basic well-being tools when I was growing up, and it was catching up to me.

That's when I discovered the breath. And I know what you're thinking: "Why does somebody have to discover breathing? Isn't that something you already know how to do?" Well, yes and no. Obviously, you know to breathe because here you are breathing and you're alive. But you see, when we experience everyday life, get into the workforce, have relationships and kids, and experience stressful moments—such as deadlines, a slew of emails, and maybe even a pandemic—we tend to hold our breath without even knowing it. In the short run, it's not that bad if you're holding your breath. You'll be fine. But in the long run, over sustained periods of constantly not giving your body the amount of oxygen it needs, overexerting yourself, stressing your natural healing systems, and energetically stagnating yourself, there are long-term and incredibly harmful consequences.

For me, I was dealing with health consequences for a while. Every time I expressed that I was feeling any type of imbalance, it was always dismissed by doctors as hormones or general stress, especially as a young woman in my early to mid-twenties at the time. I started to learn from my close group of friends that they also experienced a lot of these same symptoms that were always dismissed. We were just trained to get used to it, deal with it, or worry about it later, when we had time, instead of really looking at the roots of why we're experiencing what we're experiencing. We were essentially asked to get used to the fact that we sleep poorly, are anxious and stressed, have pain and physical ailments, experience mood swings and irregular cycles, and so much more.

It's such a normal practice to dismiss these conditions with young people. Why don't we have teachings on wellness and well-being? Why aren't we taught practical ways to make it through such common symptoms faced by so many? When I think about it even further, I'm not really sure that our caretakers, however amazing and incredible they are, had the knowledge of the super easy holistic techniques that we'll cover in this breathwork guide that can literally change people's lives.

When I first experienced the benefits of breathwork, it was a shock to my system. You mean to tell me there are breathwork techniques that can help me sleep better so that I don't have to stay up for two days at a time feeling insane? You mean to tell me there are breathing techniques that I can use when I'm right about to have an argument with someone that can help me get out of that butt-hurt mode? You mean to tell me there are techniques to heal generational pain just by breathing? You mean to tell me there are breathing techniques that I can use to energize my body when I'm experiencing chemical depletion from the shifts of the seasons and I don't have to feel like I can't get out of bed? You mean to tell me there are ways to improve my mood just by changing the way that I breathe?

Sign me up right now!

This is the exact reason I'm energized to put together this breathwork guide. This is for all of you who have ever gone through very common imbalances and were asked by society to roll over and accept them.

You are probably living just like I did back in the day. You're likely not going to make it into an hourlong breathwork class. You probably never even heard of breathwork. Meditation terrifies you. You're probably rolling your eyes at many of the woo-woo and wellness practices that you see all over social media. I get you, because I am you, and I work with people just like you.

This is the guide for all the times your partner has come home stressed-out with anxiety and cannot sleep at night. This is the guide for your parents who are old school and think meditation and mindfulness is a voodoo practice. This is the guide for teachers who have rowdy kids in the classroom with so much energy and they're punished for it. This is the guide for the nurses who want to help their patients relax. This is the guide for therapists helping clients be less anxious and more aware. This is the guide for your aunties and uncles who wear insomnia on their sleeve like a badge. This is a guide for your crabby friends who just need to take a deep freaking breath. This is the guide for everyday people just like you who are doing the best you can and are open to being a little bit more at peace with yourself. You feel me?

My friends and family around the world have started to participate in my virtual Breathwork Club—a silver lining of the digital world—and experienced the life-changing breathwork techniques firsthand. They inspired me to share these techniques in a way that was relatable, usable, and valuable in everyday life. It's truly an inspiration to see even the micro-vibrational shifts that have taken place after learning a few practical breathing tips.

Of course, my breathwork practitioners, current and former breathwork students, and clients have also informed which breathwork techniques I'm sharing in this guide. They really let me know what kind of techniques our communities are actually craving and what will be useful in an applied way. Nothing complex. Nothing too serious. Nothing that requires four years of expertise. These are real-life breathwork techniques for everyone.

My hope is that you'll be able to learn these practices not only for yourself but also for those around you. I hope that your students, parents, kids, clients, patients, masterminds, and much more will be able to benefit from these super-easy, usable techniques that I honestly believe everyone should have access to at any age.

And if you think you're bad at meditating or feel intimidated by it, don't worry; this guide is exactly for you. You will be able to use and adapt these breathing techniques based on the real ways in which they can be helpful for you in your life. I'll be with you the whole way.

Let's breathe,

CHAPTER

I

WHY BREATHWORK?

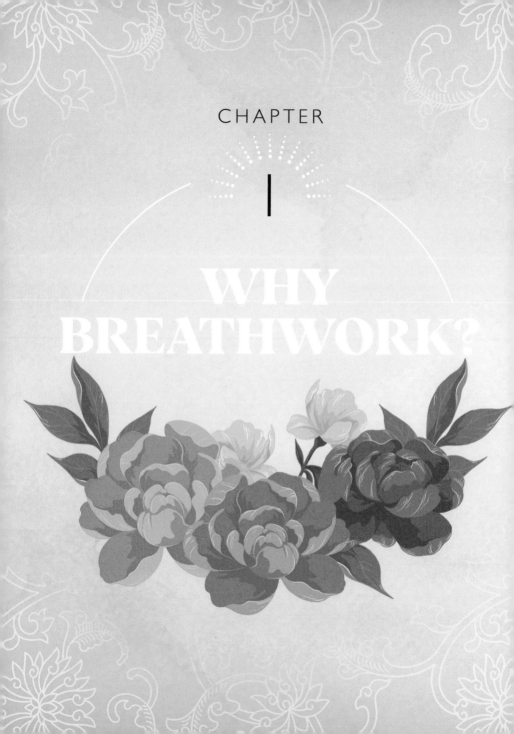

The precious gift of breath is our first taste of life when we enter this world. It is our life force. Our breath is what helps us feel calm, energized, and at peace. It supports our body's natural healing systems. It gets us into dreamland and gives us nights of deep, restful sleep. But breathing has many benefits beyond giving us life. Breathing is one of the best ways our body knows how to relax and lower our stress response. By practicing mindful breathwork, you can lower your blood pressure, better manage chronic pain, reduce feelings of depression, lower your heart rate, manage symptoms of illnesses, and much more.

By the way, I'm curious: How are you breathing right now? Take a moment to take a deep breath. When taking the deep breath, what did you do? Gasp air into your chest and puff up your shoulders? Yep, I know. In fact, most of us are holding our breath right at this very moment. We learned to become naturally poor breathers, sorry to say, and because of it, we've caused our body harm in ways we didn't mean to.

You see, our breath is more than just the air we're bringing in and out of our body. Our breath sends signals to nearly every vital aspect of our being that regulates our mood, energy, digestion, hormone production, metabolism, respiration, cell production, and so much more. When we give ourselves an opportunity to breathe, we activate the natural ways our body already knows how to support us.

It's that simple!

Cool, right?

What Is Breathwork?

So, what exactly is breathwork? Breathwork means intentionally regulating our breath. We're controlling the pace and the way that we inhale oxygen and exhale carbon dioxide. Ancient studies through the Vedas, Yoga masters, shamanic cultures, martial arts, and spiritual practices throughout the world all used the breath as a way to heal back in the day. Before we knew the science of breathing, all the different breathing techniques, and the breathwork process, our ancestors were using different styles and techniques of breathwork to energize, heal, and elevate their bodies. Ancient peoples knew that there was something about the pace, the duration, the intensity, and the rigor of breathing that changed the human experience. But at some point, we forgot how to breathe! It seems silly because obviously if you are reading this, you are breathing. And of course, you've been breathing your entire life and are doing fine so far. I get it. But the *way* we breathe has changed over time.

Think of the most expert breathers: babies. No one had to teach them to breathe; they just know how. If you look closer at *how* a baby breathes, you'll notice that they breathe into their little bellies. Trust me. If you have a baby around, go take a look. The primary deep breath they are taking is into the belly. Over time, this changes. Kids stop breathing into the belly and start to be chest breathers, just like us adults. Something happens in our life experience that switches us from these natural, intuitive, expert breathers into stressed-out breathers.

The good news is that there are plenty of tools and tips that we can use to trick our bodies into going back to the methodology that we already knew as babies. We can unlearn poor breathing.

Nowadays, breathwork is done in many different ways. Some form of breathwork is used practically everywhere—in schools, yoga studios, therapy, sports, traditional medicine, holistic healing, nursing, meditation, and trauma healing, to name a few. Here are some applied ways breathwork is being brought into the everyday community:

Teachers are adapting calming breathwork techniques and energy release techniques to bring mindful awareness to students, helping them regulate their autonomic nervous system; providing mindfulness tools to special-needs students; and promoting self-regulating breathwork during both virtual and in-person class time.

Nurses are using breathwork with patients for overwhelming and stressful circumstances, in small group meditations, in first-responder wellness programs, and with family healing.

Therapists are using breathwork with clients to move subconscious blocks that live in the body rather than the mind for somatic experiencing and somatic-based trauma healing, emotional processing, parental relationships, inner child work, and forgiveness, often in conjunction with movement-based healing techniques.

Coaches are moving away from mind-set only models and into somatic wellness to support clients in deep-level subconscious healing, emotional healing, embodiment coaching, and mind-body-spirit integration, often in conjunction with movement-based healing techniques.

Yoga studios are adapting breathwork classes that focus on several techniques for calming, energizing, connecting, and everyday use.

Breathwork facilitators are curating meditations that are in alignment with the needs of their communities: connection, spiritual and trauma healing, self-love, confidence, forgiveness, and more.

Other common practices using breathwork that we may not recognize as breathwork include:

- Singing, chanting, humming
- Dancing
- Sports
- Birthing
- Playing wind instruments
- Laughing

Can you think of other examples where your breath plays a crucial role?

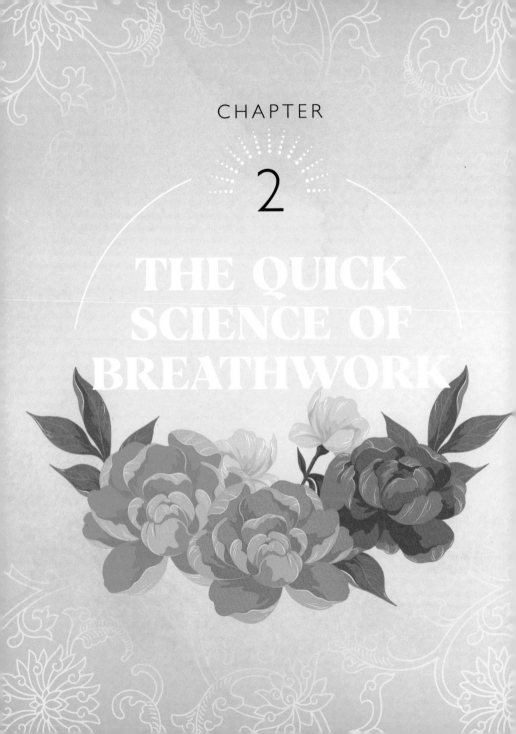

CHAPTER

2

THE QUICK
SCIENCE OF
BREATHWORK

Truthfully, you can study breathwork for the rest of your life and still not know everything. As research relating to breathwork, respiration, and consciousness continue, we are able to get much more information about all the effects different breathing styles have on us. We are only beginning to learn how breathing pace, duration, and intensity impact us on a physiological, mental, emotional, and spiritual level.

Let's cover some of the basic science of what's happening in the body when we do intentional, mindful breathwork practices. Understanding the foundations of mindful breathing will give you a much better context for how the exercises in this guide can positively impact your mind, body, and soul.

Our Nervous System

Without confusing you with an entire science course, what you need to know is that our body has something called the nervous system. The nervous system controls practically everything within our body—breathing, movement, thinking, and the way we feel. The system of nerves sends and carries messages through and to our entire body, providing information about what we're experiencing. This system also takes in what we feel and sends that information back to our brain to decipher.

Within our nervous system we have two separate systems: the central nervous system and the peripheral nervous system. The central nervous system includes the brain, brainstem, and spinal cord, while the peripheral nervous system deals with automatic responses that we don't have to think about for the most part—like breathing. This system is essentially sending information from our brain to the rest of our body.

Within the peripheral nervous system, we have two additional systems: the somatic nervous system and the autonomic nervous system. The somatic nervous system is the one that carries sensory information from your muscles and organs and is able to be controlled by you, like moving your legs or waving your arms. The autonomic nervous system is essentially all the things in the body that are automated, such as blinking, heart rate, digestion, and pupil dilation and contraction. These are all the things you don't have to think about, because your body automatically does them.

Drilling down even further, within the autonomic nervous system we have the sympathetic nervous system and the parasympathetic nervous system. I know that's a lot of systems, but stay with me here. Most of us function within the sympathetic nervous system. This is the part of us that detects whether we are in danger (or perceived danger) and activates our fight, flight, or freeze responses. When we are constantly existing in this state, we are only in survival mode. Our body prioritizes helping us survive rather than helping us thrive. Imagine being tense, nervous, and on edge all the time. I'm sure that you have felt those things at some point in your life, but imagine if that's all you were feeling all the time. You can already feel how stressed and constricted your body would be, how that tightens your chest and automatically makes you hold your breath. That's not healthy for your body, especially over time.

On the other hand, we have our parasympathetic nervous system, which essentially is our rest and restoration state. When we can lean more into this state, we help our body switch on our natural healing gears. This is like letting our body go have a cellular spa day. It gets to relax, restore, digest, bolster our immunity, and regulate our heart rate, blood pressure, and metabolism. This is the feeling you get after you've had a lot of deadlines and you finally submitted all your papers—that feeling of relief and peace that washes over you. You can physiologically feel your body switch from "go mode" to "rest mode." This is a beautiful and natural way we shift from protection vibes to relaxation vibes.

Breathwork is something that can help us switch between these two states. There's no exact transition between the sympathetic or parasympathetic nervous states because they are both active simultaneously, but we can be more in either one of these states depending on the style of breathwork we're using, along with the pace, duration, and intensity.

We also have a very special bundle of nerves called the vagus nerve that connects nearly every element of our body from our brain all the way down to our spine. This incredibly complex set of nerves is connected to our eyes, heart, intestines, spleen, and everything in between. When we do breathwork, we're activating and awakening this bundle of nerves. We're pumping oxygen and asking these bundles of nerves to work in a more optimized way. Detailed research about the vagus nerve shows long-term effects that controlled breathing can have on reducing stress, increasing alertness, and boosting the immune system. Studies have also found that breathing practices can help reduce symptoms associated with clinical diagnoses like anxiety, insomnia, post-traumatic stress disorder, depression, and attention deficit disorder. And research shows that breathwork has benefits for athletes, dancers, and others.

Breathwork techniques tend to fall into two categories: activation and restoration.

ACTIVATION

Activation styles of breathwork are the ones that—you guessed it—activate the body, bringing in energy so you feel more awake, creative, and energized. You might experience tingly sensations and an elevated mood. Activation styles of breathwork wake up the sympathetic nervous system and hyperactivate the body with tons of hormones, such as serotonin, dopamine, and even trace amounts of DMT.

This type of breathwork is amazing to do in the morning to give you a boost while you're getting ready for the day and for midday when you want an energy pick-me-up. Once you are finished with an activation breathwork practice, your body switches into the parasympathetic state, which then gives you the sensation of being at peace and at rest, even though you are filled with energy.

RESTORATION

On the other hand are restoration styles of breathwork. These techniques help calm, restore, and relax your body. After practicing restoration styles of breathwork, you'll feel peaceful, less tense, and better able to sleep.

During restoration forms of breathwork, your body goes deep into the parasympathetic state so you can rest and digest. This state is perfect for signaling to your body that you are okay and you can relax. Restoration practices are amazing for asking your body to calm and chill. For these reasons, these are great styles to practice in the midst of busy days and are perfect for nighttime.

CHAPTER

3

COMMON EXPERIENCES

As you become aware of your breath and start to practice mindful breathing, it's important to know what to expect. Emotions may come up for you as you work on your breathing and healing your body. Your body may also start to feel differently, and you may feel more connected to your inner self.

In this chapter, I share with you some of the most common experiences that can occur when practicing any form of mindful breathing. You may experience some or all of these things; you may experience none of them. You may experience something that's not listed here, and that's okay. No two breathwork sessions are ever the same, and the breath will be different for each person.

Common Emotional Experiences

It's common to have feelings come up during any mindfulness practice, and breathwork is notorious for awakening emotions that are stored in the body. Emotions are known as energy in motion and are always flowing through our body. We intuitively know that we feel emotions in certain parts of our body. For example, you might feel grief and heartache at the center of your chest. You might feel a burden right at your shoulders, neck, and upper back. You might have a gut feeling at the center of your stomach.

When you do any style of breathwork, there is a possibility that an old emotion that's been living in your body will resurface. You may also feel a resistance to a particular emotion. It might be a surprising emotion— something you were not expecting to feel. It might be a random emotion—something out of the blue. It might be something that you've been repressing that you didn't know about, or it might be something you've been repressing that you are well aware of.

If any emotions come up, I invite you to allow those emotions to show you why they're here right now. Give yourself permission to feel the thing, even if it feels uncomfortable, random, or unexpected. I also invite you to reflect, journal, integrate, and ponder why that emotion may have shown up for you. How long has it been living in your body and where are you carrying it? It can be a really powerful tool to observe that emotion and also investigate why it's showing up.

Common Mental Experiences

It's okay to have a busy mind before, during, and after any form of mindfulness practice. In fact, because we're human, it would be silly for us to expect to fully shut off our brains and thoughts. A busy mind is the exact reason why breathwork is a beautiful and transformative practice for the mind.

You might experience a busy mind as you go through the techniques in this book. You might think of your to-do lists or notice the sounds around you. You might get distracted from the practice as well. You might experience moments of stillness and observe the thoughts floating through. You might notice the sensation of calm, peace, restoration, and release. All of it is okay.

A breathwork practice isn't about shutting off our brains and having nothing to think about. It's about allowing ourselves to be mindful and intentionally in the moment. You'll also notice that certain breathwork techniques are more mentally active than others. Some will remind you that you have a lot on your mind and others will make you forget you were thinking of anything at all.

Breathing is a practice of being in the present moment. If your mind has a lot of activity at this moment, go ahead and observe that.

Common Physical Experiences

With each of these breathwork techniques you will feel something slightly different. I'll make sure to let you know what you might feel with each technique, so you know what to expect as you do that particular practice.

Overall, in most of the activation styles of breathwork, it's very common to feel tingling sensations, light-headedness, chills, goose bumps, and hot or cold temperatures. You'll feel gentleness, tension release, and other calming sensations when doing styles of breathing for relaxation and grounding. The beauty of breathwork is that changing up the pace and the style will create different physical sensations as different techniques release more or less chemicals in the body.

If any physical sensation feels alarming or unbearably uncomfortable, definitely slow down your breath or close out that practice. All the physical sensations are cues that the breath is going exactly where it needs to go and allowing your body to recalibrate. Listen to your body's cues if a certain style is not right for you.

Common Spiritual Experiences

Practicing any form of breathwork or mindfulness is a deeply integrative and connecting experience. The practice of breathwork truly connects the mental, emotional, physical, and spiritual bodies. In this process, you might feel a deeper connection to yourself, a peace in your heart, and a sense of oneness. You might feel a connection to Source Energy (a higher power), ancestors, and guides. You might feel as if you've left your body and traveled elsewhere. You may especially feel the emotional body, physical body, and mental body all blending together as one unified experience instead of three separate things.

Cultures around the world use longer forms of some of these techniques for spiritual healing, generational healing, trauma healing, and ancestral healing. It is difficult to put into words what any of those things actually feels like, but what I will say is that be open to the power and potency of what your breath can show you. Give yourself permission to surrender to your breath and the potential of what you might experience.

Allow the emotional, mental, physical, and spiritual sensations to come through as you begin developing your daily practice. Some techniques will activate certain elements more than others, meaning that some of these techniques will activate your emotions a little bit more than the physical body, or might awaken the spiritual a bit more than the mental. Be open to the possibilities, and just keep breathing.

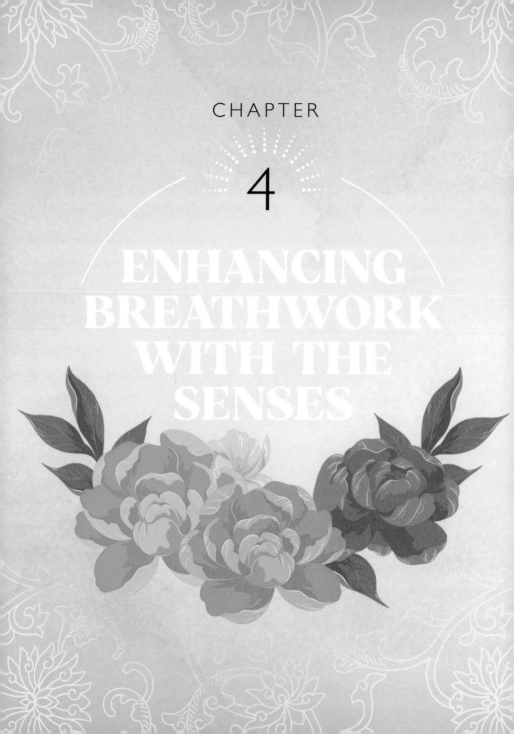

CHAPTER

4

ENHANCING BREATHWORK WITH THE SENSES

B reathing by itself is enough.

I don't want to confuse you by saying that you need all these extra elements or enhancements while you use the power of your own breath. The whole point of breathwork is that you don't actually need anything except yourself. The breath will always go where it needs to go, and your body will always direct it accordingly. However, if you'd like to add extra elements to your practice, you can incorporate other senses with your breath: visual, scent, and listening.

If you are new to practicing intentional breathing or any of the techniques outlined here, I recommend that you begin your breathwork practice without any additional enhancements and stick to practicing the techniques as they are while you're just getting started. Practice and master the techniques so that you get the feel of how each one truly feels in your body. Pay attention to what you feel physically, emotionally, mentally, and spiritually. As you get the hang of each technique, you can play around with adding other elements and combinations that complement your practice.

For each breathwork exercise in this guide, you'll find a few suggestions for what you can add to your practice. Do what feels the most natural to you. Have fun and find a way to practice that most aligns with you. You can skip all the enhancement suggestions altogether. It's really up to you. There's no wrong way to practice breathwork!

How to Use Visuals

Breathwork can be practiced with your eyes open or closed. There's no special rule about this. Sometimes when you're practicing breathwork in your daily life, you don't actually have the option to close your eyes. For example, you might be practicing a relaxation technique while you're driving, and I do not recommend that you close your eyes during that time! There are other techniques where it's quite nice to close your eyes; it gives you a better opportunity to feel more of the sensations that are passing through you and allows you to be present and mindful in a different way than if you had your eyes open. This is always a personal preference for you as an individual and how you choose to experience and practice breathwork.

There are people who like to close their eyes to go deeper inward. For some people, closing their eyes can help them focus on their breath instead of focusing on other things in the environment that can feel like a distraction. Some people close their eyes and float off into an imaginary world. Breathwork is notorious for activating the dreamland and theta states; the visualizations, colors, and downloads that come through in this state are often best experienced with the eyes closed. You might also use prerecorded guided meditations while you practice breathwork and visualize a whole environment in your mind's eye. This can be super powerful and enriching as well. Some techniques that are for relaxation and sleep are often best experienced with closed eyes.

Others like to keep their eyes open. Some people like to observe what's in the environment. They like to notice the details, the movement, and the stillness. Some people keep their eyes open and focus on a particular object or place. This can be as simple as gazing at a plant, a candle, or your hand. Sometimes visuals, graphics, and other environmental cues are used in breathwork practices as a focal point. This is also a great way to practice being intentional and mindful while being in the midst of your regular day-to-day life.

Although I'll give you suggestions on whether a particular practice is better done with your eyes open or closed, you can choose to practice all the techniques as you prefer. You can always switch it up and try it in different ways for any of the techniques. It really doesn't matter what you choose; the breath will do its job either way!

EYES OPEN

If you are practicing with your eyes open, you can try a soft gaze or a focused gaze.

A soft gaze means that you can gently keep your eyes open without really trying to look at something in your environment. It is when you aren't exactly staring at something, but you see it in your peripheral vision. For example, you aren't looking at your cat, but you see what they're up to over there. This soft focus can be incredibly powerful at times when you can't really close your eyes in the middle of a meeting, but you can definitely use that intentional breath to help you center. The soft focus is also good for helping you stay present with your breathwork technique. It allows you to be here in the NOW rather than floating off too far away from your environment to the point you forget that you were even practicing breathwork.

On the other hand, a focused gaze is when you decide you're going to look at something directly, with intention. You can pick something to look at that's already where you are, or you can bring in an object of your choice. Many people use a lit candle, flowers, or the sky. The object that you pick is less important than staying with your breathwork as you also observe with your eyes.

When you are focusing on an object, you can follow along the edges and match your breath to it. For example, if the technique asks you to breathe in for five seconds, you can gaze out your window to the tree outside and follow along its edges for five seconds; if it asks you to hold your breath for five seconds, you can follow along for another five counts through the edge of this tree, the branches, and the leaves. Notice all the beautiful details, the colors, and the textures in the meantime. Now if the technique asks you to exhale for five seconds, go ahead and finish drawing an outline around the tree until you come back to your starting point. You can use the focused gaze method for practically any object that is near you.

If you decide to practice your breathwork techniques with your eyes open, regardless of whether you practice with a soft gaze or a focused gaze, observe your environment while focusing on your breath. This means pay attention to where you are. Notice what's around you. Notice the colors, the vibrancy, the movement, and the sensations that surround you. You don't necessarily have to look at something directly in order to know that there are other things in your environment. This is a big one because, realistically, when you practice breathwork, you'll likely be in an incredibly busy environment with lots of people and things happening around you. These practical tips are for times when you're not in your Zen Den at home, the kids are screaming in the background, you don't have a quiet space with relaxing music, and you are practicing when you are in the midst of a lot of different things going on all at once.

You may also choose intentional visuals and imagery. Perhaps you want to look at a photograph, mood board, screensaver, nature, or scenery. It's up to you. You can try to create visuals in your mind's eye, meaning you can visualize a beach, park, or scene in your imagination.

EYES CLOSED

It's a little bit different practicing breathwork with your eyes closed. Having your eyes closed really allows you to be open to visuals and images that can show up in your mind that aren't concretely present in your environment. Keeping your eyes closed while practicing breathwork can also be an incredible way to receive guidance from sources that are outside of you. You might receive downloads or messages, visuals, animal symbology, and depictions of things that you weren't trying to create in your mind. You might experience colors, sensations, swirls, and much more. It can also be nice to be able to see nothing.

If you are practicing with your eyes closed, you can try one of two things. The first way is to simply close your eyes and do nothing. After the first few moments, you might start to notice the colors and lights shift, even with your eyes closed. The key here is to release expectations and release your eyes.

The second way to practice breathwork with your eyes closed is with guided imagery. Begin to imagine within your mind's eye. Where do you want to be right now? For example, let's pick a garden. Visualize the garden in your mind. What colors do you see? Notice all the little details. What are the textures? What types of lines and edges can you see? Go forward within this environment; perhaps you want to look down and see the grass, notice the flowers in the distance, and the birds in the air. You can choose to zoom in or zoom out to any part of this visualization; for example, you can zoom in on the details of the flower petals, or you can zoom out and see the garden as a whole.

How to Use Scents

Scents are another fun component to add to breathwork practices. Scents and smells have a powerful effect on activating memories, emotions, and feelings. One way to use scents is to observe the scents that are already in your natural environment, especially if you're somewhere in nature like a garden that has beautiful scents of flowers. Of course, if you're somewhere that doesn't necessarily feel like it smells good, you can skip this part.

Another way is with essential oils. Essential oils can be inhaled or if diluted with a carrier oil, be applied directly to the skin. Each way will give you a slightly different experience. When you inhale an essential oil, odor molecules travel into your olfactory receptors, swish through a few sections of your brain, then move into your limbic system, and then into your pituitary gland, where it then gets distributed to your endocrine system—your adrenal glands, thyroid, and digestive hormones. This is a faster way to experience the oil because you get an immediate effect.

If you apply essential oils topically, meaning that you put it directly on your skin, it'll have a fast path to your bloodstream but you will feel the effects less immediately; it'll go to your digestive system, respiratory system, muscles and joints, vascular system, and finally your hormonal system. Because of that, it's important to source essential oils that are of the purest natural qualities. Go for oils that don't have any additives beyond the oil and the mixer itself. You don't want to use artificial elements because they have a direct passage into your bloodstream. Even though topical application is a slower way to experience the effects of the oil, it will last longer.

Note: Always make sure the oil is diluted with a carrier oil before applying to skin, and make sure to test an essential oil on a small area of your skin before using it topically. You might want to ask your doctor before using anything on your skin.

Not all breathwork techniques will benefit from scent. Some practices are done best just by themselves without additional enhancement. I'll give you suggestions in each technique for what scents you might consider using. Here are the four essentials oils we'll be working with in this guide:

- **Peppermint** is a refreshing oil that helps open up the nasal passages and chest during breathwork. It also has calming effects, reduces stress, improves mental function, and alleviates pain. When applied directly to the skin, there's also a nice cooling and tingling sensation that feels awakening. This is a perfect oil to use with almost all techniques, especially ones that help ground and energize.
- **Cinnamon** is a super-activating oil that boosts the entire body. This oil has properties that energize mood, support cognitive function, improve memory and attention, and boost creativity. This is a great oil to use during mood-elevating and energizing styles of breathwork. It's advised to use this oil sparingly because it's quite strong and can also have an intense heat element to it.
- **Rose** is super loving and relaxing. This is a heart-centered oil that has a lot of healing properties. It helps reduce anxiety, stress, and fear. It promotes connectedness, sensuality, abundance, prosperity, and love. Rose oil is perfect for centering, inner healing, and grounding breathwork.

❧ **Lavender** is a calming essential oil that promotes relaxation, rest, and sleep. This restoration oil has properties that reduce insomnia, anxiety, and stress. It is a perfect oil to dab on during relaxation breathwork or at nighttime before going to sleep. You can also add it to your bathwater to let your entire body absorb its healing qualities.

How to Use Listening

You are welcome to practice breathwork with sound or in silence. The beauty of breathwork is that it is meant to be practiced anywhere and anytime. You do not need complete silence for any breathwork technique, or any special type of sound or music.

Practice listening. What's in your environment? What's around you right now? In busy environments, you can practice listening to the bustling sounds. Observe what you hear: the footsteps, voices, dishes, cars, birds, moments of silence, and everything in between. Even in the midst of it all, can you stay with your breath? Can you allow your body to receive these beautiful breaths without the sounds feeling distracting or overwhelming?

Music in itself is a form of meditation and adding intentional breathing to it can really change your experience. Binaural beats, lo-fi sounds, Zen meditation music, sound healing with crystal bowls, and 432 Hz frequency are all amazing for a breathwork practice. You can of course add other types of music to your practice. When beginning, it's great to pick selections that do not distract you from the breath at hand. Can you stay with the breathing technique while this music is playing? Are you so into singing the lyrics that you forgot that you were doing breathwork?

There's also no rule that you have to sit still during breathwork. As long as you are breathing, you're good to go. In fact, many breathwork classes use music, drums, movement, and dancing! I'll share a few of those in this guide. Maybe you want to listen to music that gets you moving. Maybe you want to groove to something. Maybe you'd like to sway. Maybe the stillness is exactly what your body craves. Whatever your energy is calling for, go with it.

When breathwork techniques have specific counts to it, you can pick music that helps you keep count by its beat. Music tracks can also help you commit to a time frame for your practice. For example, you can say you're playing these four songs and you'll stay with your breathwork practice until the playlist is over. This way, you're listening to something you love, and the time will pass by quickly because you're bringing breathwork goodness into your body at the same time. Of course, you can use guided meditation tracks that help you stay present and with your breath as well.

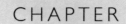

5

BREATHWORK TECHNIQUES

Now that we have the foundations down, let's get breathing. As mentioned earlier in the introduction, these practices are broken down into five categories that are easy to navigate for you: mood, energy, inner healing, relaxation and grounding, and sleep. You can choose to practice these in any order that you wish and skip any that do not resonate with you. I highly recommend trying them all out at least once, so you get a feel for them, and pick your favorites to put into your daily practice. As discussed in chapter 4, you have lots of choices available during your practice: visuals, scents, and listening.

For your first practice, keep it simple and start with Just Breathe on page 44. This is the only exercise that is not within one of the five categories I mentioned before. This simple practice is perfect for all situations.

Before you get started on your daily practice, fill out the following breathwork inventory (page 42) either in your journal or mentally and take notice of your breath. After your practice, take some time to answer the reflection questions either on a separate piece of paper or mentally.

Note: If you have a history of light-headedness, fainting, or a medical condition that prevents your participation in sustained breathing, please consult your doctor before practicing breathwork.

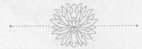

Breathwork Inventory

Complete this Breathwork Inventory before you begin each practice. Take a note of your answers mentally or write them in your journal or on a separate piece of paper. You can take a picture of the inventory on your phone so that you have it with you for times you aren't carrying this guide. You can also fold down the corner of this page to make it easier to come back to. There are no right or wrong answers to this inventory. This is just for you to be aware of your body and notice your own relationship with your breath. As you develop a consistent practice of mindful breathing, notice how your answers shift as well.

1.   **How are you breathing?**

   ❀ Through my mouth

   ❀ Through my nose

   ❀ Oops, I was holding my breath

2.   **Where are you breathing into?**

   ❀ My face

   ❀ My shoulders

   ❀ My chest

   ❀ My belly

   ❀ A combination (where?)

   ❀ I can't tell

3. Take a deep breath in. How did you breathe?

   - Through my mouth
   - Through my nose

4. Take a deep breath in. Where did you breathe into?

   - My face
   - My shoulders
   - My chest
   - My belly
   - A combination (where?)
   - I can't tell

5. About how many breaths have you taken this minute?

6. What is your intention for your practice today?

7. How are you emotionally?

8. How are you mentally?

9. How are you physically?

10. How are you energetically/spiritually?

1

JUST BREATHE

Duration: A few seconds or more

Call upon this technique anytime you'd like to:

- ⚜ Take a moment for yourself
- ⚜ Feel peace
- ⚜ Catch your breath
- ⚜ Celebrate yourself
- ⚜ Relieve stress
- ⚜ Oxygenate your body
- ⚜ Calm your thoughts
- ⚜ Gather your emotions
- ⚜ Slow down anxious responses

This breathwork exercise is designed to help you keep it simple.

I know it's really irritating when people tell you to "just breathe," but what if they were onto something? In times when you need a simple reminder to breathe, the practice of just breathing can be a game changer.

You are likely somebody who is constantly holding your breath without even knowing it. This tricks our body into thinking that we are constantly in our fight, flight, or freeze mode. It essentially believes that we're in danger. When we breathe, we signal that we're really okay and that our body can activate the parasympathetic nervous system, which prioritizes all the beautiful ways that our bodies know how to help and heal ourselves naturally.

In the daily happenings of life, you may find yourself in situations where it's not possible to take a break by yourself. You might have a lot of busyness in your mind. You might feel heavy emotions or reactive in certain ways. In times where there is a lot going on, just breathe.

Use this simple reminder to help your body get out of the fight, flight, or freeze response and into a much calmer state where you are able to act from a place of love for both you and others. This is a practice you can do on the fly without needing anything else. Even just a few seconds of this practice can bring incredible healing changes that you'll notice immediately. There's nothing to prepare, nothing to see, nothing to do. Just breathe.

THE PRACTICE

1. Sit, lie down, or stand exactly where you are.
2. Pick a number between five and ten.
3. Use the number you picked to breathe in through your mouth or nose for that number of seconds, keeping count in your mind.
4. Exhale out the same way for that number of seconds.
5. Repeat for at least ten rounds of breathing.

TIP

Don't worry about adding anything else to this technique and keep this practice as simple as possible.

REFLECTION

- What do you notice about the way you're breathing right now?
- How can you give yourself a few extra reminders throughout the day to breathe this way?

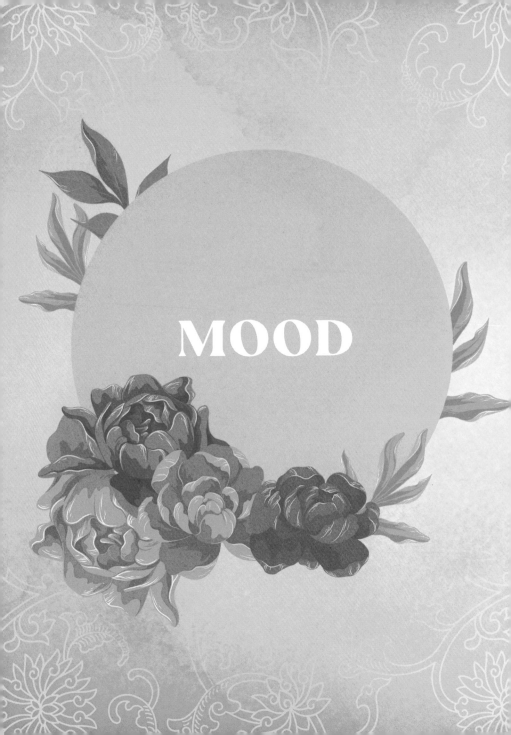

MOOD

Techniques in this section are all for elevating your mood. For times when you feel an emotional lull, don't have a lot of energy, are feeling down and out, or experiencing seasonal changes, you can use any one of the techniques in this section.

You'll also notice that many of the mood-boosting techniques have a little bit of movement to them. This is because our breath and body both dictate how we feel. When we move our body and connect it with our breath, we give ourselves access to incredible feel-good hormones that help us feel better and clear out stagnant energy. You can do these as still or with as much movement as you'd like!

2

THE LAUGHING BREATH

Duration: 30 seconds to 7 minutes

Call upon this technique anytime you'd like to:

- ❧ Increase energy

- ❧ Boost immunity

- ❧ Improve mood

- ❧ Have fun

- ❧ Connect with others

- ❧ Increase feel-good hormones

- ❧ Shake out stagnant energies

- ❧ Stretch

Let's have a laughing fit! Did you know that laughing is a form of breathwork?! Did you know that laughing has healing properties? Yes! And if you've been taking yourself way too seriously lately, this is going to be the technique for you.

Laughing has incredible benefits for us. Aside from the reason that it's fun, there are also immune-boosting reasons for why laughter is a crucial part of what keeps us happy and healthy. Laughing has the ability to trigger our immune system and regulate our nervous system. It boosts the release of endorphins that are our body's natural feel-good chemicals. So, when you laugh and you feel kind of high, it's essentially because all these beautiful hormones are being released and pumping through your body. Often, these hormones are actually sitting in our stomach doing their thing, but we aren't fully accessing them because they aren't getting pumped to the rest of our body.

Laughing as breathwork also protects our heart health. It's essentially like getting a ton of cardio that improves the function of your heart and the blood vessels that are around your heart. Laughing helps your heart get stronger because it's having to pump more blood and work harder to keep it strong.

Of course, laughing is also a mood lifter. I'm sure you know that when you laugh you're having a good time! Laughter has also been shown to reduce the stress hormone cortisol, which is responsible for making us feel anxious and tense. Cortisol is the primary stress hormone that releases from our body and our brain when we are experiencing stressful events or what we perceive as stressful events. Laughter also improves your circulation because now you don't have an overwhelming amount of cortisol circulating in your body.

Another beautiful part of laughter is that it helps you release control. Sometimes we're control freaks; we want to control everything around us. We want to know the outcome of everything. When you laugh, you kind of let go of those expectations of control and allow yourself to naturally have fun. You get to enjoy your current experience rather than thinking about the past or the future.

When you practice laughter as a breathwork technique, it's pretty common to feel like you're forcing it at first. I've definitely seen this happen quite a bit. At first when you start, it feels unnatural. It kind of feels like you are faking this experience because there might not really be something funny for you to laugh about. Maybe it feels weird to hear your own voice. However, surrender to the experience. Remember what I said about letting go of control? This is about doing the motion of laughing so that you can essentially trick your body into releasing these feel-good hormones and trick your subconscious mind to shift into the vibration of joy. We can actually feel ourselves into a better mood rather than thinking ourselves into it. In fact, studies have found that simulated laughter can be just as good as the real thing!

THE PRACTICE

1. Standing, sitting, or lying exactly where you are, put your hands on your belly and laugh like you heard something really funny!

2. Keep going for at least thirty seconds.

TIP

Try this practice in a group! Bring together your coworkers, friends, kids, and family members and just let go! You'll notice how liberating and freeing it feels to hear others also express pure joy and happiness. It'll be contagious and, before you know it, there definitely will be somebody rolling on the floor laughing like a hyena!

REFLECTION

- How often do you laugh during the day?
- How do you feel about the sound of your laughter?
- How did your laughter change as you kept up with it?

THE GODDESS BREATH

Duration: 3 minutes

Call upon this technique anytime you'd like to:

- ❀ Elevate mood
- ❀ Feel inspiration
- ❀ Feel empowered
- ❀ Increase energy
- ❀ Increase feel-good hormones
- ❀ Improve digestion
- ❀ Improve respiration
- ❀ Inspire confidence
- ❀ Improve posture

Call upon the Goddess Breath when you're ready to totally shift your entire mood. Goddess energy is all about confidence, elevation, motivation, and embodying how powerful and potent you are. It exudes a self-assured aura and inner potency. This energy holds both love and conviction. The goddess is the one bringing both gentleness and power.

But of course, you don't always feel self-assured. Maybe you're down and out. Maybe your self-confidence is not really the best lately. Maybe you're exhausted. Maybe you're not getting the proper chemicals and hormones flushing through your body. Maybe the weather has been changing and you haven't felt like yourself in a while. Whatever it is, you can use this breathwork to bring in empowerment and embody goddess energy.

Give yourself plenty of space to move for this practice. You're calling in your superpowers and embodying a royal energy, so go ahead and envision yourself as this incredibly expansive energy that's not afraid to take up space. Throw your shoulders back, put your head up, align your gaze, relax your body, give your arms the ability to move freely, and claim this energy for yourself.

Here's the thing: oftentimes your mood is impacted by the way that you carry your body. When you hold your body very constricted, small, and hunched over, you're sending energetic signals to yourself that you are essentially afraid to be seen right now. Anytime you send signals that you are either not worthy of being seen or you're afraid to be seen, it impacts the way you feel. This can manifest in your everyday life by how much interest and energy you have to do regular activities, by the excitement you have behind your projects, by the creative downloads that you receive toward your art and businesses, and so much more.

With this breathwork, you're going to send the exact opposite signals to your energetic body and remember that you have a lot of creative portals within that you always have access to. This breathwork reminds you to command your space and your energy as you connect your body to your movements, your breath, and your personal energy. So even if you might not actually feel super empowered or embodied when you start, this breathwork is going to help you embrace that vibe more.

What you may experience during the breathwork is a sense of awakening. This breathwork is well known for awakening any kind of energy that has been stagnant within the body. You might feel a bit light-headed, tingly, and energized. Physically, you'll experience the feel-good hormones pumping through your cells, improving your respiration, digestion, and, of course, your overall mood.

Move your teacups and laptops, and take up that space.

THE PRACTICE

1. Stand or comfortably sit on the ground or on a chair (standing is recommended).

2. Begin to visualize your whole body (or at least the upper half of your body if you're sitting) moving in a circular motion. Start the first breath from the bottom of the circle and move your body forward in a circular motion through each step.

3. Take a quick breath through your nose as if you're reaching to breathe in air at the bottom of the circle and then take this breath into your full body without exhaling between the two inhalations.

4. Take another quick breath through your nose and rotate your body to the top of the circle.

5. Exhale out of your mouth almost forcefully, making a "HAAAA" sound on the exhale as you close the circle at the bottom and squeeze out from your belly.

6. Repeat for at least ten full rounds of breath without pausing in between the inhales and exhales. If you'd like to do this breathwork for longer than three minutes, it's recommended that you practice with a trained facilitator that can support you through the intensity of this practice.

TIP

Do this breathing exercise in front of the mirror and add empowering music. See yourself moving through the powerful energy within your body. Notice what it feels like to see yourself reclaim and activate your energy. Notice your posture. Notice your gaze. Look at yourself. Have fun with yourself and embrace how powerful you are.

REFLECTION

- What did it feel like to make big sounds?
- How did you feel moving your body?
- How did you feel seeing yourself during this breathwork?

4

THE STRAW BREATH (3-3)

Duration: 30 seconds to 7 minutes

Call upon this technique anytime you'd like to:

- 🌿 Increase energy
- 🌿 Increase feel-good hormones
- 🌿 Improve digestion
- 🌿 Improve respiration
- 🌿 Improve focus and concentration
- 🌿 Release stagnant energy
- 🌿 Relieve stress

The Straw Breath is a perfect way to neutralize any stagnant energies within the body. This is a great one to do just as you're getting started for the day or for those times when you're having a slower morning and could use a pick-me-up in your mood.

What our body wants to do is have an equivalent amount of oxygen going in at the same rate that carbon dioxide releases out. Often, we're taking in too much oxygen and not exhaling enough carbon dioxide. Other times, we are holding our breath, so we have a lot of carbon dioxide in the body but not enough oxygen. It's all about balance. So, the Straw Breath is one of the best ways to equalize how much oxygen is coming in and the rate of the carbon dioxide going out. The practicality of using this breath is that you don't need to have a lot of preparation to do this practice. The key to this breath is to keep your inhalations and exhalations the same pace, duration, and intensity.

It's pretty common to feel light-headed after a few rounds of this breath. So, if you have any history of fainting, panic attacks, vertigo, or previously known light-headedness from taking quick breaths, this won't be the right technique for you. Also, it's not recommended for kids to do this method of breathing for any prolonged period of time. They can absolutely do it for up to five rounds but not any longer than that.

THE PRACTICE

1. Sit or stand comfortably upright.
2. Take three medium sips of air in through your mouth as if you were sipping water through a straw.
3. Blow out at the same pace three times from your mouth as if you were blowing out of a straw.
4. Repeat for a few rounds all the way up to seven minutes.

TIP

If you've got one around, it's fun to use an actual straw for this breathwork technique. You can physically put a straw in your mouth as you practice this one. The size of the straw doesn't matter; it's just the fact that you are puckering your lips a certain way in order to receive an equivalent exchange of air coming in and out. Reusable straws are perfect for this practice!

REFLECTION

- What was it like taking consistent sips of air in and out?
- What sensations did you experience?
- How did you maintain a consistent pace?

5   THE STRAW BREATH (6-6)

Duration: 30 seconds to 7 minutes

Call upon this technique anytime you'd like to:

⚜ Increase energy

⚜ Increase feel-good hormones

⚜ Improve digestion

⚜ Improve respiration

⚜ Improve focus and concentration

⚜ Release stagnant energy

⚜ Relieve stress

This variation of the straw breathwork has the same philosophy and benefits as the one right before this technique (page 55). In this variation, you'll take in more sips of air and exhale for longer as well. Because you're taking longer breaths, the effects of the breathwork is going to be quicker and more intense. This short burst of oxygen often goes directly to the head and it's common to feel extra light-headed with this technique. The key to this breath is to keep your inhalations and exhalations the same pace, duration, and intensity.

This is not the right practice for you if you have a history of fainting, panic attacks, vertigo, or previously known light-headedness. Also, it's not recommended for kids to do this method of breathing for any prolonged period of time (five rounds max).

THE PRACTICE

1. Sit or stand comfortably upright.
2. Take six short sips of air in through your mouth as if you were sipping through a straw.
3. Blow out short bursts of air six times from your mouth as if you were blowing out of a straw.
4. Repeat for a few rounds all the way up to seven minutes.

TIP

Use your listening senses for this technique. Listen to the sounds and lengths of your inhales and exhales. Use the sound to help you keep the pace consistent.

REFLECTION

❀ What was it like taking consistent sips of air in and out?

❀ What sensations did you experience?

❀ How was this similar or different from the Straw Breath (3-3)?

THE STRAW BREATH (6-3)

Duration: 30 seconds to 7 minutes

Call upon this technique anytime you'd like to:

- 🌱 Increase energy
- 🌱 Increase feel-good hormones
- 🌱 Improve digestion
- 🌱 Improve respiration
- 🌱 Improve focus and concentration
- 🌱 Release stagnant energy
- 🌱 Relieve stress

This variation of the Straw Breath also has a similar philosophy and benefits to the ones right before it (pages 55 and 58). In this variation, you'll take in quicker sips of air through your mouth, but elongate the exhales this time.

As with the previous techniques, this is not the right practice for you if you have a history of fainting, panic attacks, vertigo, or previously known light-headedness. Also, it's not recommended for kids to do this method of breathing for any prolonged period of time (five rounds max).

THE PRACTICE

1. Sit or stand comfortably upright.

2. Take six short sips of air in through your mouth as if you were sipping through a straw.

3. Slowly blow three long exhales from your mouth as if you're blowing out of a straw, pausing briefly between each exhale.

4. Repeat for a few rounds all the way up to seven minutes.

TIP

Play around with which part of your body you are breathing into to sustain the longer breaths. Try breathing into both your belly and your chest to create more space for the oxygen.

REFLECTION

✻ What was it like blowing out slowly this time?

✻ What sensations did you experience?

✻ How was this similar or different from the other Straw Breaths?

THE CHANTING BREATH

Duration: 7 minutes or more

Call upon this technique anytime you'd like to:

- Relieve stress
- Recalibrate vibrationally
- Invite in relaxation
- Connect to self
- Calm your thoughts
- Release nervousness
- Release tension in the neck and shoulders
- Improve concentration and focus
- Slow down anxious responses
- Rest your energy

Chanting is an age-old healing practice and, as it turns out, also a form of breathwork. Many religions and spiritual practices around the world have chanting, mantras, and gospels as an integral part of their practice. I'm sure that you've seen monks, choirs, prayers, or some form of religious chanting in your lifetime somewhere. You may have practiced chanting without even knowing so.

Aside from the religious and spiritual experience of chanting, and the repetition of prayers and mantras, in breathwork, there are some very amazing benefits for the everyday person. Research has shown that long periods of chanting can change the brain's chemistry. Prolonged chanting helps synchronize the left and right brain hemispheres and reduces stress, anxiety, and other tensions that can manifest from energetic imbalances. Chanting can also help you get into deep flow states where you feel like you are "in the zone." If you play music, sing, dance, write, or create anything, you understand what that flow state is. It's that feeling when everything is flowing out of you. You're downloading information and your creativity is just pouring out. That flow state is also a deep restorative meditative brain state that activates your body's natural ability to heal itself. This theta brain state is between consciousness and unconsciousness; it's often described as being in a dreamworld.

Chanting helps you stay in that flow state while you also experience the ultimate rest, where your parasympathetic nervous system kicks into high gear; here, you get all the benefits of traditional meditation without being a seasoned expert.

Chanting is also a form of vibrational healing. The actual sounds that come out of your mouth when you chant, even if you think they sound odd, are healing for the body. As you exhale, you'll feel a vibration from the sound you're making. This vibrational element has the power to help recalibrate anything in the body that's vibrating too fast and boost what's underactive.

If you ever found yourself singing the chorus of a song over and over again, or repeating a saying, chances are you have done some form of chanting in your life. In fact, I'm sure that at some point you were cheering for a sports team and chanting cheers at teammates! The act of making sound from your throat has a cathartic effect. However, this Chanting Breath is less about exact words or a particular sound, tone, or formation. It's more about the action of chanting itself.

THE PRACTICE

1. Lie down, sit, or stand as you feel comfortable. Having a comfortably upright spine is a great choice.

2. Breathe in through your nose into your full body (belly and chest).

3. With your mouth open, make an audible long "ahhhhh" sound until you are out of breath. You can play around with the sound on your exhales. You can say ah, ee, iii, oh, or oo. It's up to you. You can also change the pitch, volume, or tone.

4. Repeat as many times as you like.

TIP

You can use peppermint oil right at the throat for a cooling effect in this powerful energy center of the body.

REFLECTION

- What do you notice about your voice?

- What does it feel like to hear yourself?

- Did the sound and strength of your tone change as you practiced?

8 · THE GULP BREATH

Call upon this technique anytime you'd like to:

- ✤ Elevate your mood
- ✤ Increase energy
- ✤ Quickly oxygenate the body
- ✤ Catch your breath
- ✤ Feel inspiration
- ✤ Increase metabolism
- ✤ Increase digestion

The Gulp Breath is another fun way to wake up your body anytime you're feeling low in energy, lacking inspiration, or want to activate creativity or elevate your mood. The Gulp Breath is exactly what it sounds like. You will be gulping air into your body!

When you try this breathwork, you'll also notice that it feels very similar to gasping. Do you know why we gasp? We gasp when we are surprised, yes, but it's essentially a natural way for your body to get more oxygen when your fight, flight, or freeze response has been triggered. We gasp as a natural response because our body automatically goes into a constricted protection mode that limits the flow of oxygen.

Gasping also helps activate a few very cool natural survival mechanisms. For example, when you gasp, the pupils of your eyes start to dilate so that you can see better. This is a way for our eyes to bring in more light for us to see predators. Your metabolism rate will also increase because this quick burst of oxygen is now fueling your muscles in case you have to run away really fast. Being scared also naturally makes us want to hold our breath. Anytime you're tense, nervous, or anxious, it's a very natural thing to stop fully breathing. You take a big gasp in to remind yourself to keep sending oxygen to your brain so that you can stay alive. Do you recall anytime recently when you've gasped?

You might also know that we may gasp when we cry. You probably have gasped while crying at some point! Our body has a tendency to go into hyperventilation when we cry to release emotions and energy. During these times, our body's automatic response is to give us more oxygen by force. Hence, we often gasp when we are ugly crying!

THE PRACTICE

1. Sit or stand comfortably.
2. Gulp or gasp a big breath of air in your lungs very quickly through your mouth.
3. Close your mouth and exhale through your nose, almost from the back of your throat, for at least four seconds, or until all the air in your body is out. This will feel like you're keeping a big passage open in the back of your throat and you'll hear the exhale from your throat even though you are exhaling out of your nose.
4. Repeat at least seven times.

TIP

Sounds have a very powerful vibrational healing component, especially when they're coming from our own body. On the exhale through your nose you can try to hum "hmmmm." This will also help the exhale come from the back of the throat rather than from your nose.

This is a super fun exercise to do with a bunch of kids or a big group. As you can imagine, everyone going "hmmmm" can be fun, connecting, and mood-boosting. See how long you can extend these exhale sounds together.

REFLECTION

❀ Where in your body did you feel this breath?

❀ What did you feel after the exhales?

❀ How long can you extend these exhales?

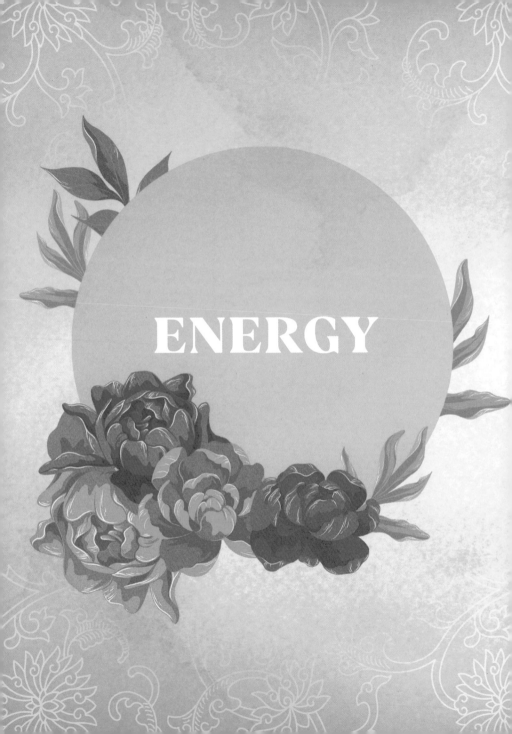

ENERGY

Techniques in this section are all for uplifting your energy. These are the practices you want to call upon when you're feeling low energy or need to focus, find inspiration, or shake out stagnant energies—especially if you've been sitting all day. All of these practices are super fun and are created to help you feel more free!

Energy-boosting breathwork techniques tend to be activating; these will definitely keep you up if you practice them at nighttime or before bed. Use these techniques earlier in the day so you can truly benefit from the energy boost. You can keep peppermint and cinnamon oils handy to use with any of the practices in this section. It's also recommended that you hydrate and replenish the fluids in your body even more than normal after energy-boosting breathwork.

THE FLUTTER BREATH

Duration: 30 seconds to 7 minutes

Call upon this technique anytime you'd like to:

- ❖ Increase energy
- ❖ Increase feel-good hormones
- ❖ Improve digestion
- ❖ Improve respiration
- ❖ Improve focus and concentration
- ❖ Improve mood
- ❖ **Release stagnant energy**
- ❖ **Relieve stress**

The Flutter Breath, or the Breath of Fire, is an activation-style breathwork used in many yogic practices. This rapid way of breathing in and out of the nose both silences and energizes the body, pumps up feel-good hormones, reduces the stress response in the sympathetic nervous system, activates the rest responses in the parasympathetic nervous system, and improves overall respiration. That's a lot! This go-to breathwork is a crowd-favorite morning practice to both bring bursts of oxygen into the body to wake up and to exhale out stagnant energies from the night before.

During the Flutter Breath, short bursts of inhales and exhales are taken in through the nose while pumping the belly in and out. This pumping motion also improves digestion, releasing the serotonin in the gut and toning the abdominal muscles. As the body receives all the feel-good hormones, it's common to feel energized, slightly high, out of your body, and focused.

For this breathwork technique, it's also common to feel light-headed and dizzy. You may experience visuals, lights, and shapes. When first starting out with this practice, do this technique slowly for a short period of time and increase your pace and duration as you improve.

If you have any history of fainting, panic attacks, vertigo, or previously known light-headedness from taking quick breaths, this won't be the right technique for you. It's also not recommended for kids to do for any prolonged period of time. If you decide to practice this for more than seven minutes as a beginner, it's best to do it with a professional facilitator.

THE PRACTICE

1. Sit comfortably with your spine as naturally upright as possible.

2. Place your palms facing up in receiving mode on your lap or knees.

3. Close your eyes. You can choose to roll your eyes up and inward toward your forehead.

4. Take a short, quick breath in through your nose as you puff up your belly.

5. Exhale out quickly through your nose as if you're blowing something out of it and squeeze in your belly.

6. Remove any pause in between the inhale and the exhale.

7. Speed up the breath so that the full motion of the breath going in and out sounds and feels like the quick fluttering of hummingbird wings.

8. Keep the movement in your belly connected with the breath: let it go out on the inhale as you fill up with air, and let it come back in on the exhale. Listen for your breath going in and out and keep up the rhythm.

9. Unclench your jaws and relax your forehead.

10. Repeat for at least thirty seconds.

TIPS

Place a few drops of peppermint or cinnamon essential oils on your palms, below your navel, on your lower back, above your heart, or in between your eyebrows on your third eye.

Since this breath is super activating, it's easy to get tired after a few seconds. This is a great one where a playlist or a soundtrack of music can help you stay in this practice for a sustained period of time.

REFLECTION

❀ What was it like to hear your breath loudly today?

❀ What was it like to connect the movement of your belly to your breath?

❀ What did you experience emotionally, mentally, physically, and spiritually?

THE PUFF BREATH

10

Duration: 30 seconds to 7 minutes

Call upon this technique anytime you'd like to:

- ⚘ Increase energy
- ⚘ Increase feel-good hormones
- ⚘ Improve digestion
- ⚘ Improve respiration
- ⚘ Improve focus and concentration
- ⚘ Release stagnant energy
- ⚘ Inspire creativity

The Puff Breath is another activation-style breathwork that's used to energize the body. This breathwork technique pumps feel-good hormones throughout the body, brings in big bursts of oxygen, and helps move away stagnant energies that are still sitting in your system.

Think of this breath as "huffing and puffing." At first try, this breath might honestly feel a little chaotic! This is because anytime you've naturally done this breathwork without even knowing it, it was probably because you did something really strenuous and you were totally out of breath! This is also something you naturally do when you have a really good cry. You know what I'm talking about—that feeling when your body is contracting by itself and it almost feels uncontrollable. It's that sensation when it almost feels like a desperation to catch your breath rather than something that's meant to be helping you.

However, your body does this breathwork naturally when you've done something

physically difficult because it's trying to provide your body with the necessary oxygen and remove the excess carbon dioxide that has collected. During the Puff Breath, big bursts of inhales and exhales are taken in through the mouth while pumping both the chest and belly in and out. This pumping motion signals to your body to wake up, reenergize, and optimize your lung capacity to receive oxygen. The huffing and puffing is the natural way you calibrate.

As the body receives the big bursts of oxygen and all the feel-good hormones, it's common to feel energized, out of the body, light-headed, and activated. A few minutes afterward, it's common to feel very creative and focused.

If you have any history of fainting, panic attacks, vertigo, or previously known light-headedness from taking quick breaths, this won't be the right technique for you. This is also another exercise that is not recommended for kids to do for any prolonged period of time.

THE PRACTICE

1. Sit comfortably or stand with your spine as natural as possible.

2. You can choose to keep your eyes open or closed.

3. Relax your arms however it feels comfortable, or place one hand on your belly and another on your chest.

4. Take a quick puff of breath in through your mouth into your entire body as if you're out of breath. You can feel both your belly and your chest rise with this. Be mindful of breathing into the belly and chest rather than into your shoulders.

5. Exhale out your mouth as if you are puffing out a sigh of relief. You may feel your entire body release tension.

6. Your exhales can be slightly longer than your inhales.

7. Remove any pause in between the inhale and the exhale.

8. Focus on keeping this breath at a consistent rate rather than trying to speed up your breathing.

9. Repeat for at least thirty seconds.

TIP

Place a few drops of cinnamon or peppermint essential oil on the palms of your hands and rub them together. When placing your hands on your chest and belly, you can feel the heat from the cinnamon or the tingling from the peppermint.

REFLECTION

- ⚜ Are there times when you've unintentionally done this breathwork?
- ⚜ In what ways do you feel energized?
- ⚜ Where in your body do you feel activated?

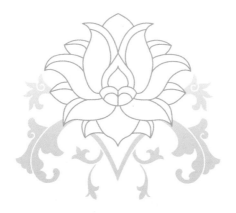

THE LION'S BREATH 1

Duration: 30 seconds to 7 minutes

Call upon this technique anytime you'd like to:

- ❧ Increase energy
- ❧ Relax muscles
- ❧ Energize the body
- ❧ Improve mood
- ❧ Feel empowered
- ❧ Increase feel-good hormones

Lion's Breath, or Simhasana Pranayama in Sanskrit, is an empowering and energizing breathing practice that is frequently used in yoga. The lion's vibration is a powerful and empowered energy; this breathwork technique helps you call that into the body while also releasing tension in your face, chest, upper back, and abdomen.

Just as lions do, the Lion's Breath is about roaring out and being in your power. It's about owning your voice. It's about taking ownership of your personal energy. While you do this breath, notice how you feel the energy shift in your shoulders, how your posture changes, how your head rises, and how your face reaches up to the sky as you take claim of this energy.

You might feel resistance to making some of the big roaring sounds that this technique suggests. That's because this technique helps activate your voice—the communication center right in the middle

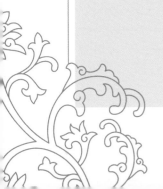

78

of your throat. This is the space where you feel empowered to express yourself and communicate authentically.

We've all been in a place where it's hard to express ourselves. Let's face it: it's not always easy to advocate for our needs and desires. That's exactly why this Lion's Breath is so important for us. It activates our communication center so that we can use our voice to speak up and be heard.

You will also notice the difference in your exhales as you continue your practice with the Lion's Breath. In the beginning, you might find a hesitation to actually make the physical sounds. You might feel shy about roaring or making any kind of noise that doesn't sound pretty. You might judge yourself about the way that you sound. But with a little bit of practice, you'll start to notice how much your communication center is craving to be opened and wants to be cleansed and cleared out. You'll even find a little bit of cooling sensation moving to the throat and the chest area.

THE PRACTICE

1. If you are familiar with the Lion's Pose in yoga, you can get into that position, or simply sit comfortably where you are, keeping your eyes open.

2. Softly gaze at the tip of your nose or directly in front of you at eye level.

3. Put your hands on your knees with your palms pressing down on your knees.

4. Take a deep breath in through your nose.

5. Open your mouth and stick out your tongue like you are trying to reach your chin with it.

6. Squeeze your throat muscles and say a long "HAAAAA" as you exhale out your mouth. You can make the sound with the air that's coming out or with your actual throat.

7. Repeat at least seven times.

TIPS

This breathwork technique can also be fun to do with music. You can choose music that has drumming or a beat that really helps you tap into the embodied and primal lion's roar.

To intensify this experience, place a few drops of cinnamon essential oil right at your throat, your heart, and two to three inches above your belly button. You can also put a drop on the back of your neck.

REFLECTION

✤ What does it mean to embody the lion's energy for you?

✤ What sensations did you feel in your body?

✤ What did you experience physically?

THE LION'S BREATH 2

Call upon this technique anytime you'd like to:

- 🌿 Increase energy

- 🌿 Relax muscles

- 🌿 Energize the body

- 🌿 Improve mood

- 🌿 Feel empowered

- 🌿 Increase feel-good hormones

This variation of the Lion's Breath on page 78 has the same philosophy as the one in the previous exercise, except now we are adding another component—movement. We're adding movement because it helps attune to that lion power. The first variation helps us flex our king of the jungle muscles, but this one is the energetic embodiment of the strength and power that the lion energy brings. The lion represents courage, personal strength, loyalty, and power. The lion is a fighter in the face of obstacles. And just like the lion, you've been through so much—the challenges, the obstacles, the hardships. Now you are ready to embrace this incredibly powerful lion vibration within every single cell of your body.

As you add this movement piece to the Lion's Breath from the previous practice, notice how different this one feels. Notice how much more empowered and embodied you are. Notice how your breath and your body are connecting to the movement. Notice how you're opening your chest and your shoulders

even wider. You might also notice your voice get a little bit stronger, clearer, and more sure of itself as you continue with this practice.

As you bring the lion's energy into your body, start to envision what it would feel like to take this energy and carry it with you in your day-to-day life. How can you show up in your everyday activities feeling embodied, confident, and in your power? What would it feel like to carry this posture with you? How would it feel to roar and be seen as you are?

THE PRACTICE

1. If you are familiar with the Lion's Pose in yoga, you can get into that position, or simply sit comfortably where you are, keeping your eyes open.

2. Softly gaze at the tip of your nose or directly in front of you at eye level.

3. Put your hands on your knees with your palms pressing down on your knees.

4. Take a deep breath in through your nose and lean your upper body back.

5. Open your mouth and stick out your tongue like you are trying to reach your chin with it.

6. Squeeze your throat muscles and say a long "HAAAAA" as you exhale out your mouth and snake your body up almost as if you were licking water off the ground, like a lion. You can make the sound with the air that's coming out or with your actual throat. This will feel like drawing a big circle with your body.

7. Repeat at least seven times.

TIPS

There is no rush to this practice. Try slowing down your breath and really tuning in to your primal energy. Try speeding up your breath and embracing the rush.

Play music in the background that makes you feel like you're in the jungle, or go out into nature to practice.

REFLECTION

❧ How was this different from Lion's Breath 1?

❧ What did you notice about your body during this practice?

❧ Did you feel any temperature shifts?

13

THE ENERGY SHAKE BREATH

Duration: 30 seconds to 7 minutes

Call upon this technique anytime you'd like to:

- Increase energy
- Relax muscles
- Energize the body
- Feel joy
- Improve mood
- Increase feel-good hormones
- Shake out stagnant energies
- Stretch

The Energy Shake Breath is a fun and easy, kid-friendly technique that helps increase energy, relax muscles, energize the body, improve mood, get those feel-good hormones pumping through your body, shake out stagnant energies, and stretch. It does so many things at once—and you get to have fun!

The body loves movement—not just because it feels good to stretch but also because it helps release energy-boosting hormones that fuel your muscles, improve your mood, and aid your digestion. I'm sure you've always heard "diet and exercise" is the key to great health. But sometimes you don't want to or can't exercise, and sometimes your nutrition isn't that fantastic. Sometimes you've just been sitting at the office or chilling on your couch. It's okay. That's why we have this breath.

You can use this breathwork as an easy way to release anything that just doesn't need to sit in your body anymore. If you haven't moved a lot lately, you might be holding emotions all over your physical body. Emotions can find a home in your shoulders like a burden, as pain and heartache in your chest, as blockages in your creativity that's sitting in your belly, as tightness in your hips, and the list goes on and on.

Anytime you have pent-up emotion or energy, there is an intuitive desire to shake it out of you. You know those times you got really mad at somebody and you just wanted to shake them? Or you were so upset that your body shook? Or you got chills and shivers down your spine? These are ways your body naturally shakes.

A lot of animals use shaking as a recalibration method too. Nobody had to teach animals how to shake, but they intuitively know that it helps them somehow. Shaking is a way to recalibrate the energetic bodies as well. In fact, we intuitively know that too.

A lot of shamanic cultures have ritualistic shaking ceremonies. These ceremonies help people release stagnant energy and let go of anything that isn't being processed by the body. Drumming and singing usually accompany shaking rituals.

Although I won't be sharing any rituals with you, I'll show you how to do an energy shaking breathwork technique that can really revitalize you extremely quickly and efficiently. The nice thing about this technique is that you don't have to stand up to do it. You can be sitting in your office chair, waiting at a traffic light, sitting outside at the park, or wherever. Just give yourself room so you can shake, shake, shake!

THE PRACTICE

1. You can do this practice in any position that feels right; however, standing is recommended.

2. Breathe in through your nose as you raise your hands to the sky.

3. As you exhale, breathe out through your mouth six to ten times and say quick "has" as you shake your arms and body as if you are shaking water off of you. When making those quick "ha" sounds on the exhales, you can say them silently to yourself or quietly under your breath, or make big, loud sounds as you exhale and shake. You might notice that you start one way and adapt your technique as you continue.

4. Optionally, shake your arms from side to side. Shake your shoulders. Jump up and down. Feel free to really move your body on those exhales in any way that feels right.

5. Bring your arms all the way down as you finish the exhale.

6. Repeat at least seven times.

TIP

Play some music! Get wild with it and play something that pumps you up. What do you want to shake to?

REFLECTION

- ❧ Did you feel any resistance or judgment about shaking and making noises?

- ❧ How did you feel afterward?

- ❧ What thoughts did you notice?

14

THE WARRIOR BREATH

Duration: 4 minutes

Call upon this technique anytime you'd like to:

- ❋ Increase energy
- ❋ Improve confidence
- ❋ Release stagnant energy
- ❋ Inspire creativity
- ❋ Release tension
- ❋ Relieve stress
- ❋ Improve concentration

This breathwork technique is very similar to the Goddess Breath (page 51) and Lion's Breath (pages 78 and 82) energy. We are awakening a primal warrior source within our energetic bodies. This practice will elevate your mood, confidence, energy, and creativity and release tension at the same time. It's a powerful breathwork technique to use when you're about to go do something that feels brave—maybe you're about to give that big presentation, go on stage, make a transitional step in your life, or do something that feels incredible expansive. Call upon the Warrior Breath technique to embrace and embody a powerful, confident you.

This technique is also powerful for transmuting stagnant energy or what feels low vibe into more uplifting energy. Think about a warrior—they are ready, prepared, confident, and grounded. Envision what this grounded warrior energy would feel like, and as you breathe, take in the vibration of this warrior energy; as you exhale, let your breath take with it what you no longer need for the next version of your life.

Warrior Breath is also incredible for manifestation for this exact reason. You get to intentionally call in the things that you want and feel the energetics of what it would be like to have them. With every breath, you're breathing in with conviction. With every exhale, you're transmuting and letting go of whatever you don't need anymore. It could be thoughts you don't need, feelings you don't want, energies you no longer want to carry with you, behaviors or attitudes that don't serve you, or anything that feels old and not what you want to cultivate in the next chapter of your life.

This warrior energy is about cultivating resilience in your life as well. Resilience means you are able to go through challenges and pick yourself up even when things are difficult. The warrior lives within all of us. It's the fighter. It's the part of us that maybe isn't always dealt the perfect hand but still knows how to make the most of it.. It's the part of us that knows how to survive and thrive at the same time. It's the part of us who is doing the best we can, and here we are, we're okay. We are strong, resilient, and brave.

When you do the first inhales of this breathwork technique, take this breath into your chest—really pop up your chest and expand your rib cage just as a warrior would display their bravery. You can also look to the animal kingdom for this type of courage, such as birds that puff up their chests and throw back their shoulders to put up a brave front when defending their nest. And even though we aren't necessarily defending something physical and we're not actually trying to fight anybody or anything with the Warrior Breath, we are essentially declaring our presence. We are here, and we are breathing.

THE PRACTICE

1. Sit or stand with your feet planted firmly on the ground and your hands by your sides.

2. Keeping your eyes open for this practice is recommended.

3. Breathe in quickly through your nose as if you're taking in a big shot of air and feel your chest fully puff up. You're not breathing into your shoulders, but you will feel an expansion there.

4. Exhale forcefully out of your mouth as if you're blowing a piece of paper away from you. Feel your chest deflate.

5. Repeat this cycle seven times.

6. Then hold your breath for thirty seconds.

7. Repeat the whole practice seven times.

TIPS

Create a playlist of songs that feel empowering and energizing to you. You might also want to use a mirror while you're practice this. This way, you get to see what it looks like to embrace the warrior energy. What does your posture look like? How are you carrying yourself? How do you feel embracing and embodying a warrior?

REFLECTION

❧ How did your stance and movement change from the beginning to the end of your practice?

❧ What did you notice in your body?

❧ What does it mean for you to embody warrior energy?

15   THE STARFISH BREATH

Duration: 30 seconds to 7 minutes

Call upon this technique anytime you'd like to:

- <small>❁</small> Increase energy
- <small>❁</small> Release stagnant energy
- <small>❁</small> Relieve stress
- <small>❁</small> Stretch
- <small>❁</small> Release tension
- <small>❁</small> Improve concentration

The Starfish Breath matches the regenerative properties of the sea star, holding the energy of personal space, vigilance, action, and intuition. When your personal energy or space feels compromised, call upon this breath to neutralize the chaos around you and center back to your natural expression. In this breathwork, you will be channeling in those vibes as you improve your mood, increase energy, relieve stress, stretch, and awaken your own intuitive body.

Most likely when you think of a starfish, you picture a rigid and tense sea star chilling at the bottom of the ocean. They're not moving; they're not doing much. These beautiful creatures like to mind their own business and love spending time in their own company. They're independent, still, and more complex than meets the eye. That might be you too!

You might be someone who loves to be in your own company and truly appreciates the peace and serenity of your personal space. Perhaps you love surrounding yourself

93

in an environment that feels safe and supportive. But we all know how it goes—there's always something or someone up in our personal space! This could be when something is physically or energetically in your personal space. It's that feeling when you know someone is overstepping their boundaries or projecting their opinions onto you. It's that feeling when you come home and you're carrying the energy of the day on your body. It's that feeling when someone shares something heavy, and a dense metaphorical cloud starts to collect around you.

The Starfish Breath is about cleansing and neutralizing that energy. Starfish carry very fluid and quick movements within their tiny bodies even if they are classic chillers; they have hundreds of tube-like feet that give them the ability to move quickly and intentionally with calculated agility. These tiny tube feet can pop out at any moment and let the starfish move and change its space—just like that.

If you are heavily connected to your intuition, you know when your personal space is compromised energetically. It can happen sneakily, and it can happen over time. When you become aware that it has happened, call in this breathwork technique to shift the energy swiftly. And as this technique is about reclaiming your energetic space, you'll want a little bit of moving space for this practice.

THE PRACTICE

1. Standing is recommended for this one.

2. Closed eyes are recommended for this practice.

3. Breathe in through your mouth and raise your arms out to your sides like a starfish.

4. Breathe out of your mouth for five quick puffs as you pump your arms down on each puff.

5. As you move your arms, feel the energy around you neutralizing. You can do this as quickly or as slowly as you'd like.

6. Continue for at least seven rounds of breathing.

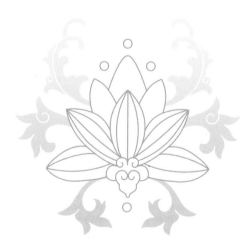

TIP

Keeping your eyes closed, visualize a golden ball of light around your body as you bring up your arms. On the exhales, visualize this light clearing and cleansing the energy around you. Let this light help you reclaim your personal space and energy. You are also welcome to move around in your space and bring your arms in front of you as you do this practice.

REFLECTION

✤ How does it feel to spread your arms out like a sea star and feel ownership of your space?

✤ How does your personal space feel different afterward?

✤ Can you practice this more slowly next time?

16   THE CANDLE BREATH FOR ENERGY

Duration: 30 seconds to 7 minutes

Call upon this technique anytime you'd like to:

- ❋ Increase energy
- ❋ Release stagnant energy
- ❋ Relieve stress
- ❋ Improve concentration

This breathwork technique is very similar to the feeling of blowing out candles or a match. You take a deep breath in and then blow air out as if you're trying to help your younger sibling put out the birthday candles on their ice cream cake without them knowing what you are doing. This means you've got to put a little extra umph behind that blow so it can reach those candles without you having to be right in front of their cake. You feel me?

This is another fun technique you can pull out of your tool kit whenever you want to move stagnant energy out of your body. This is a good one if you sit all day for work or tend to be a couch potato. The motions will activate your chest and belly at the same time. When you're sitting so much, there tends to be a lot of energy that collects right at your gut.

If you're sitting down while reading this book, you probably already intuitively feel that there's a little bit of energy collected right there in your tummy. This stagnant energy can create pain in the lower back and give you a hunchy posture. Your gut flora—the microbiome that supports your immune system, blood sugar, cholesterol, and much more—has a lot to do with your overall health and well-being. If you don't move enough, all these juicy chemicals and flora keep sitting right there in the center of your belly. As they just sit and chill, the rest of your body would love to have access to the benefits of this goodness.

You probably intuitively already do this practice without knowing it. When your body and energy feel really tight, it's likely that you've been holding your breath or breathing only from your chest. You're not getting enough oxygen, friend, and your body is collecting carbon dioxide that has no business being there.

What's really fun about this technique is that as you blow out those metaphorical candles—or real candles, if you want to use them—you're also letting out a sigh of relief. And that's exactly how you want to treat this breathwork: you are releasing energy and liberating your body. You also let go of any tightness in your shoulders and chest and release any emotional burdens that have been stagnating in you. You awaken your belly and your gut flora, and that's a huge relief. Feel yourself letting go.

THE PRACTICE

1. You can practice this technique in any position.
2. Breathe in through your mouth.
3. Blow out air from your mouth as if you are blowing out a candle.
4. On those inhales, breathe into the belly and chest at the same time so you're filling up most of your body with air at once.
5. On those exhales, squeeze your belly in so that you are releasing all the air from your body at once.
6. Repeat at least seven times.
7. You can play around with the length and intensity of both your inhales and your exhales.

TIP

You can enhance this practice by using actual candles. Be careful when using fire and do not leave flames unattended. You can also visualize candles and practice the strength of your breath on the flame.

REFLECTION

- How does it feel to hear yourself sigh?
- How do you intuitively sigh during your day?
- Is there a difference practicing this with your eyes closed versus opened?

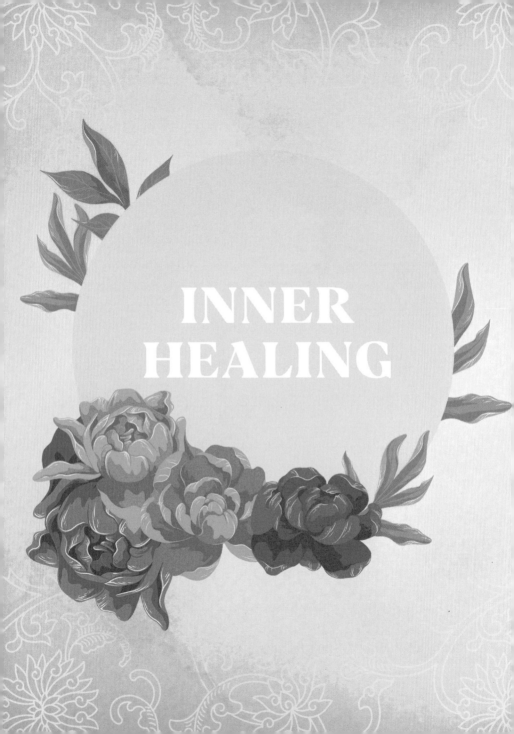

INNER
HEALING

n the section, you'll find several techniques that are meant for inner healing. If you're on a self-healing journey, in the midst of spiritual exploration and personal development, there'll be a few breathwork techniques that you'll want in your tool kit.

Many inner healing techniques are best experienced with a certified breathwork facilitator and those who hold intentional space for inner healing to take place. It's great to have a facilitator and a support system because inner healing techniques can often bring a ton of emotions and energies that require deeper integration afterward. When done with a qualified practitioner, these techniques can bring on life-changing and transformative experiences. People have described it as twenty years of therapy after just one session! They are some of the world's greatest somatic healing tools.

THREE-PART BREATHING
TECHNIQUES

Three-part breathwork is a profound breathing technique that is used for energy healing, vibrational alignment, recalibration, subconscious healing, grounding, and self-love. The three-part breath is also known as a circular breath because you are breathing in a circular motion. This breath first comes into the belly, awakening the stagnant energies and emotions that sit here, travels to the chest, opening up the heart, and exits fully in a circular motion.

I highly recommend that you do not try to do the techniques in this section for longer than the recommended duration. It's perfectly safe for you to use these techniques by yourself if you are using them briefly according to the directions outlined here. For any longer practices, you 100 percent want to have a certified breathwork facilitator who can see you through your journey with care.

These techniques are not recommended for kids or for those who have any prior respiratory issues, history of vertigo, heart problems, or blood pressure concerns.

17 THREE-PART BREATH (NOSE)

Duration: 3 minutes

Call upon this technique anytime you'd like to:

- ❀ Bring in inner healing
- ❀ Access self-love
- ❀ Boost energy

In this variation, the full breath is done through the nose. Generally, try breathing into your belly through your nose a few times and then try it with your mouth. Do you notice the difference of how much air your body is able to take in and how deep or shallow the breath is with your nose versus your mouth? Where do you feel it when you breathe in through your nose versus your mouth? Where is the air going? What are the sensations?

The experience of doing this breath through the nose means that there are quick injections of air into the center of the body and the head.

THE PRACTICE

1. Lie down as flat as possible with nothing under your head or your lower back.
2. Closed eyes are recommended for this practice.
3. Place one hand on your belly and one hand on your heart.
4. Take a deep breath in through your nose into your belly and feel your hand move as your belly fully expands.
5. Without exhaling, take another breath into your chest, feeling the hand on your chest expand. Keep your shoulders still.
6. Exhale out your nose longer than both inhales took and feel your body fully empty out.

TIP

You may feel yourself rushing through the breaths in this practice. Listen to the sound of your breaths and create a consistent pace.

REFLECTION

- What sensations did you experience?
- What thoughts floated through?
- How did it feel to breathe into both your belly and your chest?

18 THREE-PART BREATH (MOUTH)

Duration: 3 minutes

Call upon this technique anytime you'd like to:

- ❧ Bring in inner healing
- ❧ Access self-love
- ❧ Boost energy
- ❧ Oxygenate the full body
- ❧ Improve respiration

This technique is going to feel a little bit different than the previous one through your nose (page 103). With every breath in through the mouth, you're bringing more oxygen into the body. You're expanding your energetic body and activating your sympathetic nervous system a little more quickly than you are when breathing in through your nose. Even though it's a very similar technique, the sensations are completely different. As you breathe through your mouth, you might also get a dry mouth, chapped lips, and a dry throat. It's okay, and that's normal. Make sure you drink a ton of water after you do this particular exercise. Prolonged mouth breathing in your everyday life is also not recommended. When you catch yourself breathing through your mouth all the time, notice why your body is asking for air in this way.

THE PRACTICE

1. Lie down as flat as possible with nothing under your head or your lower back.

2. Closed eyes are recommended for this practice.

3. Place one hand on your belly and one hand on your heart.

4. Take a slow, deep breath in through your mouth into your belly and feel your hand move as your belly fully expands.

5. Without exhaling, take another slow breath into your chest, feeling the hand on your chest expand. Keep your shoulders still.

6. Exhale out your mouth longer than both those inhales took and feel your body fully empty out.

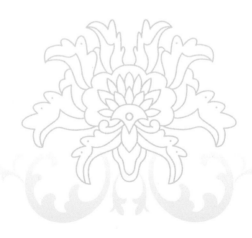

TIP

Create a short "calming" playlist with your favorite soothing sounds and use this playlist as you practice this breathwork to help you further bring your mind to a place of peace and tranquility.

REFLECTION

- How was breathing in through your mouth different than breathing in through your nose?
- What sensations did you experience?
- What did you notice about your energy?

19   FLOW BREATHWORK

Duration: 3 minutes

FLOW Breathwork is the ultimate form of full body somatic healing. This is my own unique blend of the three-part breaths we practiced in the last two exercises combined with studies of martial arts, Ayurveda and the elements, movement, energy healing, and dance. Call upon this breath when you are ready to reclaim the power within yourself, activate your intuition, and fully come into flow in every aspect of your life.

Being in flow is to be in unity with your vessel—your body and your breath. To be in flow is to harmonize with the Universe. To be in flow is to trust.

Often, we try to become in flow by force. We try to follow rules and regulations for how and what healing looks like. We try to limit what our body already naturally knows how to do and feel. We try to overintellectualize what flow even means. We are constantly looking outside of ourselves for healing, but not at what's already inside of us.

But of course, forcing flow, though tempting, is counteractive. Flow is unique to you and how you are integrating what's going on around you. It's those times when you are so tapped into your projects or conversations and your creative juices are flowing. It's when you are writing and the words just come out by themselves. It's when you're singing, and you get lost in the song. It's those times when you feel like you're being guided by something outside of you, and within you at the same time. Things feel easy—almost too easy! You are resting *and* activated. You are centered. You are in *flow.*

In this practice, imagine yourself as an instrument in an orchestra, meant to harmonize with what's around you. Your thoughts, reactions, actions, behaviors, environment, and social settings are all notes in the song. How is your instrument tuned to be in harmony with them? Is what's around you in dissonance with what you feel within?

And how do you flow with the elements that you exist in? Earth, water, fire, air, and ether are all around you as well, bringing in different energies of grounding, ease, activation, freedom, and expansion respectively. Is there too much fire in your body that leads you to burn out? Is there an imbalance in air that stagnates creativity? Is there over-grounding that prevents you from joy and play?

To flow, is to bring back balance.

As you practice the FLOW Breathwork, I'd love for you to really tap into what flow actually means for you. You will also notice how primal this particular technique feels. There is a certain softness and power to what FLOW Breathwork brings: a freedom and a rhythm. This breathwork helps balance the masculine and feminine energies within the body. Often, when we are too heavily within either masculine or feminine energy, we feel a mood imbalance. We feel that we are out of our element. Come back to center. During this breathwork, what we're essentially doing is a full recalibration of both these energies. There's a powerful strength and reclamation as well as a sensual softness.

Give yourself plenty of space to move for this practice. Feel free to channel in the elements as they feel relevant for you. Feel free to lean into the way your body wants to express during this practice. And most of all, have fun!

THE PRACTICE

1.   Stand up with your feet planted on the ground.
2.   Snake your body in a circular motion for a few rounds before you start the breath. Allow your body to loosen and relax.
3.   On the next circle, breathe in through your mouth at the bottom of the circle.
4.   Take another breath through your mouth as your body comes to the top of the circle.
5.   Exhale through the mouth slowly, and intentionally as you squeeze the breath out of your body and begin to close the circle.
6.   As you get into the rhythm of connecting your body and breath, start to move your hips, ribs, and arms in a way that feel natural to you, while keeping the breath pattern. You can also play around placing your hands on your body in a way that feel intuitive.
7.   Repeat for at least three minutes. If you'd like to do this breathwork for longer than three minutes, it's recommended that you practice with a trained facilitator that can support you through the intensity of this practice.

TIPS

Practice this in front of the mirror. It is also highly recommended that you practice this breathwork with music that helps you feel like you're present in your body. You might even want to try to experiment with humming or singing through a flow breathwork practice.

REFLECTION

🌾 Where in your body did you feel resistance?

🌾 Where in your body did you feel ease?

🌾 How did it feel to connect your breath to your body?

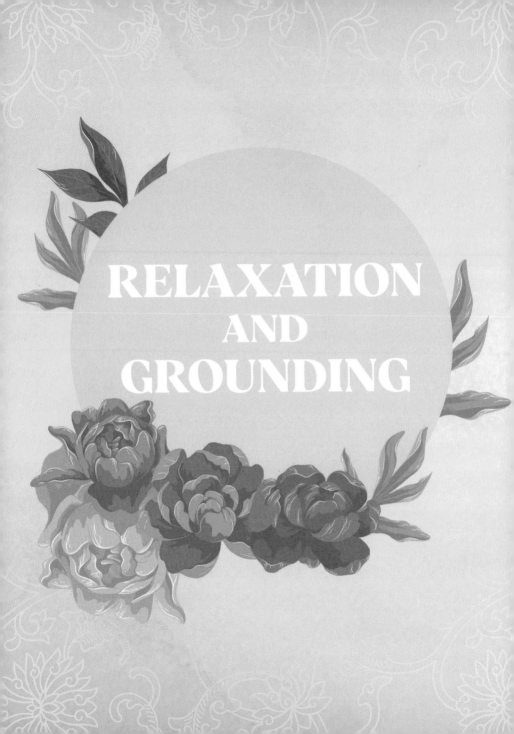

RELAXATION
AND
GROUNDING

n the section, you'll find breathwork techniques that are incredible for bringing in relaxation and helping you stay grounded. Many of these techniques are super easy for kids and can be done in a few seconds. Relaxation and grounding techniques are all about helping you come back to your body in the midst of a busy and active day. For times when you want to ground your energy, ease tension, reduce stress, relax your muscles, and feel rest and relaxation, pick a breathwork technique from this section.

Relaxation practices are all relative to what helps *you* feel relaxed. Do you prefer a particular environment? A soundscape? Your pets nearby? Sunlight? Moonlight? A cozy nightie? Whatever it is, many of these techniques can be practiced in the environment that invites the most amount of relaxation for you.

There are also techniques that help recreate that relaxation feeling for times you can't really get away and create or be in the environment of your choosing. You can essentially trick your body into feeling grounded and centered. Let the breath guide you.

THE BOX BREATH

Duration: 2 to 7 minutes

The Box Breath is a powerful relaxation breathing technique that slows down the body's automatic responses and activates the parasympathetic nervous system to help bring in peace and relieve stress. This is a great technique to call upon when you're feeling overwhelmed or want a minute to catch your breath. This technique brings in oxygen intentionally, slows down overactive thoughts and feelings, and returns you to a state of rest.

When practicing this breath, imagine a box.

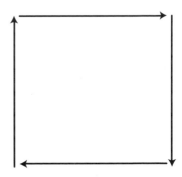

This box represents how you will follow along with your breath. Starting at the lower left corner, you'll inhale up the left vertical edge, hold your breath across the horizontal top edge, exhale down the right vertical edge, and hold your breath on the horizontal bottom edge back to your starting point. This allows your mind to slow down while giving you an activity to focus on by drawing the box in your mind's eye. You'll notice that all the chatter in your mind will ease, you'll start to feel relaxed almost immediately, and you'll also almost forget what you were thinking about. This is a powerful technique to refocus yourself. If you have a lot of mind chatter, this technique can help you refocus.

The nice thing about this breathwork technique is that you can do it in the midst of a really busy day, in between meetings, during meetings, while prepping your kids' lunches, and so much more. This technique is really powerful to do with your eyes open, and it's a great practice to call upon when you're not able to close your eyes.

If you don't have this breathwork guide available and you want to do this technique, you can look at anything that's a square, rectangle, or a shape with four sides, such as a window, book, laptop screen, or mouse pad. You can do this breathwork with your eyes closed as long as you can visualize a box in your mind's eye.

This is also a powerful technique when you are feeling really overwhelmed. When there's a lot of activity happening around you—the kids are running around, the traffic is really loud and hectic, and you're in the middle of juggling and managing all these life activities—the Box Breath is the perfect reset.

THE PRACTICE

1. Sit or lie comfortably.

2. Keeping your eyes open for this exercise is recommended.

3. Look at the box on page 114 or imagine a box in your mind if your eyes are closed.

4. Breathe in for five seconds through your nose following the vertical line up the left side of the box.

5. Hold your breath for five seconds, following the horizontal line across the top of the box.

6. Exhale for five seconds through your nose, following the vertical line down the right side of the box.

7. Hold your breath for five seconds following the horizontal line across the bottom of the box.

8. Repeat at least five times.

TIPS

As your body's ability to receive and hold the breath increases, you can play around with the timing of your breaths and holds. Try it out using six seconds, eight seconds, and so on. Notice what feels right for your body and take it from there.

The visual piece of this practice is different from many other breathwork techniques. Play around with seeing a box physically on the page, looking at a window, or envisioning it in your mind's eye. Another way to practice this box technique is to physically draw a box on a piece of paper. The repetitive motion becomes meditative, gives you a task to focus your mind, and has an amazing relaxation effect.

REFLECTION

- ✤ What was it like to use a visual with your practice?
- ✤ What did you notice about your thoughts?
- ✤ What was it like to practice holding your breath?

21

THE 6-7-8 BREATH

Duration: 7 minutes

Call upon this technique anytime you'd like to:

🌿 Relax

🌿 Relieve stress

🌿 Calm your thoughts

🌿 Improve sleep

🌿 Improve concentration and focus

🌿 Slow down anxious responses

We've all been there; we've all had those super-hectic days where it feels impossible to find a moment to ourselves. We're doing so many different tasks that we actually forget to breathe. For those days when you are taking care of everyone else but yourself, do this breathwork technique just once or twice and you'll notice a huge difference in how you feel afterward.

I also highly recommend showing this technique to your kids, parents, students, and clients because of its potency and how easy it is. Essentially, we're breathing in a pattern that slows down our sympathetic nervous system, which makes us feel like we are in the fight, flight, or freeze mode. We then activate our parasympathetic nervous system, which helps us feel a little more at rest even if it's just for a few seconds.

Those few seconds over time can be crucial to our overall health. Overexertion can harm our digestion, immunity, hormone regulation, and even information processing.

We aren't getting enough oxygen through our system that allows us to rest so that we can optimize our body, and instead, we're using up precious resources that can really tire us out in the long run.

The 6-7-8 Breath slows down the body in just a few seconds. It invites calm, focus, and re-centering and lets your body know you aren't in danger.

THE PRACTICE

1. Stand, sit, or lie down just where you are.

2. Breathe in through your nose for six full seconds, counting down in your head: 6-5-4-3-2-1.

3. Hold this breath for seven seconds, counting down in your head: 7-6-5-4-3-2-1.

4. Exhale out your mouth for eight seconds, counting down in your head: 8-7-6-5-4-3-2-1.

5. Repeat for as long as you'd like.

TIPS

If you'd like to add music that feels right for you in the moment or something that helps you keep count, you are invited to add that to this practice.

You can also place a few drops of a calming essential oil, such as lavender, on your palms, rub them together, and bring them a few inches from your face as you inhale throughout this practice.

REFLECTION

❧ Listen to the sounds of your breath entering and leaving your vessel.

❧ What differences do you notice after this practice?

❧ Did you find yourself rushing through any parts of this?

22

THE DIVER'S BREATH

Duration: Up to 7 minutes

Call upon this technique anytime you'd like to:

- Relax
- Relieve stress
- Calm your thoughts
- Increase oxygen in the body
- Release tension
- Improve concentration and focus
- Slow down anxious responses
- Rest your energy

Do you ever wonder how scuba and free divers can hold their breath for so long underwater? Well, it's breathwork and it's all about practice! You see, most of us are chest breathers, meaning that when we breathe, we take oxygen into our chest instead of our belly. Breathing into all parts of our body, both the belly and the chest, increases the reserve of oxygen we have and removes carbon dioxide at the same rate. If we aren't removing carbon dioxide at the same rate our body produces it, then our body and brain will ask us to breathe faster and essentially signal to us that we are suffocating.

Sometimes even when we're not trying to hold our breath underwater, we replicate this feeling of suffocation in our daily lives. This can manifest as feeling extra anxious, tense, and nervous. This feeling can happen as we're sitting in our office chair waiting for a meeting, feeling anxious or nervous about something, or anticipating a stressful event. Our bodies have a natural inclination to put us in this suffocation mode.

The Diver's Breath is a super-slow technique that brings oxygen into our body by gradually breathing into our belly and the lower third of our lungs. Then, we breathe into our chest and into our full lungs. This process of slowly allowing air to enter the body at this intentional pace increases our capacity to hold and maintain oxygen over time. The slow place of the exhale allows the body to learn to exchange carbon dioxide and oxygen at an ideal rate.

When first practicing this technique, you might find yourself rushing. The key here is to slow down the inhale as much as possible. Over time, you'll notice that your body's capacity to breathe in air slowly will increase.

THE PRACTICE

1. This technique is best practiced seated in a comfortable upright position. You can also lie down for this.

2. Puckering your lips as if you are drinking from a medium-size straw, breathe super slowly from your mouth into your belly and feel your belly expand all the way out.

3. Without exhaling, bring this inhalation all the way into your chest and feel your ribs and chest expand all the way out.

4. Exhale out your mouth the same way.

5. You can do a few rounds of this or all the way up to seven minutes.

TIPS

Play around with how long and slow you can maintain these inhales and exhales. Remember, divers do this breath to increase their lung capacity and reduce the use of their oxygen tanks underwater. They want to take the least number of breaths but make the most of each one. You'll notice that your capacity to both breathe in and out will change even after a few rounds of doing this breath.

Sounds of the ocean or water can be a powerful tool with this breathwork. Find a playlist that has sounds of gentle waves or streams that you can use when doing this technique. You can also place peppermint essential oil on your upper chest and throat area to help open up the passage of air. The cooling sensation from the oil will be a nice effect as your breath capacity increases over time.

REFLECTION

- Listen to the sound of the breath. Does it sound like the ocean? Waves?

- Did the breath in feel longer or shorter than the breath out?

- Did you notice a change of how long you could breathe in and out after a few rounds?

23

THE HUMMING BREATH

Duration: A few seconds to 7 minutes

Call upon this technique anytime you'd like to:

- Relieve stress
- Recalibrate vibrationally
- Invite in relaxation
- Calm your thoughts
- Release nervousness
- Release tension in the neck and shoulders
- Improve concentration and focus
- Slow down anxious responses
- Rest your energy

The Humming Breath, or Bhramari Pranayama in Sanskrit, is an incredibly beautiful way to bring absolute peace and calm to yourself. It's named after the buzzing or humming sound that's made when you exhale during this breath. The simplicity of this technique is what makes it so accessible for everyone. This is a popular one for kids to practice and something you can do together even when there's a lot of noise around you.

This breathwork technique also has a very special element to it: vibrational healing. In the Humming Breath, when you exhale you keep your mouth closed and make a buzzing or humming sound. While you do this, your body experiences a very special vibration. As you know, vibrations have the power to heal us; everything within us is constantly vibrating. Sometimes things within our cellular body are vibrating a little too fast and are overactive; sometimes things are a little underactive and vibrating too slowly. When we initiate this vibration on purpose, with the power of our breath, we're essentially recalibrating our vibrational body. This is almost the same effect that cats have when they purr. Research has found that there's also a very specific tonal quality and frequency in a cat's purr that lets them recalibrate their entire system. When they rub against on you, the vibration is healing you too!

Although we know less about the exact frequency humans emit when we hum, and there's less research about the exact recalibration that's happening, we still feel a vibrational realignment as we practice this breath.

Another special quality about the Humming Breath is that you feel it in your throat when you actually hum during the exhale. The humming essentially clears energy that is often collected in the neck and throat. If you've been having a hard time expressing yourself, speaking up, being heard, or using your authentic voice, this is a great cleansing breath that awakens and activates the throat center.

When first starting this technique, you might feel that your face, throat, neck, shoulders, ribs, and below your rib cage are holding a lot of tension. After a few rounds of this breath, you'll start to notice that your exhales get longer, and you will feel tension releasing from your body. A humming sound is also a cathartic release. It's almost like sighing out the tension that sits on your shoulders, neck, and chest.

What's really fun about this breathwork technique is that you can play around with the humming during the exhales. You can hum a high pitch tone and notice where in your body you feel the vibration; try humming at a middle pitch tone and see the difference in that. Lastly, try humming a really deep sound to notice where the vibrations are going now. You can also go from high to middle to low to middle to high to low to middle or wherever you want because that's the fun part of doing this breath. Over time, you'll notice the change in your tone as well as the strength in your hum.

The entire process of this beautiful hum helps calm down every single nerve you have. Many yogis and meditators use the Humming Breath when slowing down for the night. It's popular for Yin Yoga, a style of yoga that is all about resting and breathing. You can call upon this breath when you are really nervous too. Because this breath helps loosen and activate your throat, this is the perfect practice right before you're about to give a presentation.

THE PRACTICE

1. Sit or stand with a comfortable straight spine.
2. Closed eyes are recommended for this practice.
3. Breathe in through your nose into your full body for at least five seconds.
4. With your mouth closed, hum as if you are saying "hmmmmm" until you are out of breath.
5. Repeat as many times as you like.

TIPS

Try this practice with other people. The collective humming sound has a super healing effect on the nervous system in the same way that chanting does.

A tingly peppermint oil or calming lavender oil dabbed on the front of the throat can elevate this technique as well.

REFLECTION

❀ Does the strength and tone of your hum change over time?

❀ Did you exhale all the way through?

❀ Where in your body do you feel the humming vibrations?

24

THE ALTERNATE NOSTRIL BREATH

Duration: A few seconds to 7 minutes

Call upon this technique anytime you'd like to:

- Relieve stress
- Invite in relaxation
- Calm your thoughts
- Release nervousness
- Improve concentration and focus
- Slow down anxious responses
- Rest your energy
- Cool your body

The Alternate Nostril Breath, or Nadi Shodhana in Sanskrit, has a powerful way of relaxing the body and mind all at once. This technique sends a larger amount of oxygen to the body than regular breathing and helps soothe nerves.

Throughout the day, you're naturally switching which nostril you're breathing through every two to four hours, so your body naturally switches into this technique whether you're aware of it or not. However, consciously doing the Alternate Nostril Breath can recalibrate and calm you. Over time, it has also been shown to improve cardiovascular and respiratory function, balance heart rate and blood pressure, and aid in hormone regulation. This yogic breathing technique is also popular with athletes because it helps improve respiratory endurance while playing intensive sports. Because this technique activates the parasympathetic nervous system, which is all about rest and restoration, you may feel a sense of overall well-being. It also helps keep your olfactory senses open and alert.

This technique sends oxygen to different parts of your brain. When you're breathing into the right nostril, you're sending an oxygen boost to the left hemisphere of your brain. Alternatively, when you're breathing in through your left nostril, you're sending an oxygen boost to the right hemisphere of your brain. Because of this crossed connection, you might feel that you are able to focus more after you do this technique. This is because now your entire brain has received an equal amount of oxygen, which is sometimes harder to do when you're breathing regularly and not controlling which nostril is taking in or releasing air. Constricting air flow on one side helps moisten and warm up oxygen before it enters your body, and each nostril gets to essentially recalibrate and rest its filtration system.

THE PRACTICE

1. Sit comfortably with your spine upright.
2. Closed eyes are recommended for this practice.
3. Place your left hand on your left knee and bring your right hand to your nose.
4. Exhale fully out of your nose before you begin.
5. Using your right thumb, close your right nostril and inhale through your left nostril.
6. Immediately close your left nostril with your index finger and open the right nostril to exhale out through that side.
7. Then inhale from the right nostril, and use your thumb to close it.
8. Open the left nostril, exhale, and close it.
9. This is one full cycle. Continue for at least seven full rounds of breathing.

TIPS

Try not to rush and definitely take full breaths in and out as you do this practice. You're essentially inhaling and exhaling from the same nostril each turn. Focus more on getting complete breaths rather than speeding through which fingers need to go where.

Use peppermint essential oil for an energizing, cooling, and invigorating effect. Use rose essential oil to help you stay in the present moment and connected with the breath.

REFLECTION

❧ What did it feel like to breathe in and out of just one nostril?

❧ What does it feel like to breathe in through both nostrils?

❧ What sensations did you feel during this practice?

25

THE GROUNDING TOUCH BREATH

Duration: A few seconds to 7 minutes

Call upon this technique anytime you'd like to:

- Ground yourself
- Recenter your energy
- Connect to the Earth
- Come back to your body
- Relieve stress
- Invite in relaxation
- Calm your thoughts
- Release nervousness

We've all felt ungrounded before. Even when nothing is really wrong, it's possible that you don't really feel connected to your body or connected to your energy. This can manifest in your life as you being easily distracted, overthinking and ruminating, worrying, feeling out of touch or reactive, feeling nervous, not sleeping well, feeling tired all the time, and even having physical pain.

When we ground ourselves, particularly by using our breath, we're allowing ourselves to be present and come back into our body. We are taking ownership of our personal energy, helping ourselves recalibrate that personal energy, and transmuting it into something that we feel good about owning.

Lineages of martial arts all around the world have extensive knowledge about the energies that are around us and how to flow with, transmute, and neutralize the energies that we exist within. Many martial arts techniques also use a deep understanding of the breath to work with grounding energies.

In this technique, we're going to be calling upon the help of Mother Earth and energetically connecting to the healing powers that Earth can provide us. Nature has so many different healing properties—the sound of birdsong and the ocean, the colors of the sky and the sea, and the feeling of the earth beneath our feet are all healing. Time in nature has been shown to reduce stress and anxiety, improve sleep, boost overall mood and well-being, and increase connection to self and spirit.

Many of us, in the hustle and bustle of our everyday lives, have forgotten that we are part of nature too. We ebb and flow with the seasons. We need sunlight, fresh air, rain, the vibrational recalibration from the sounds of nature, and all the beauty Earth provides.

For any number of reasons, many of us don't spend a lot of time outdoors. When you can't get out into nature, use this technique to access a feeling of groundedness. If you are able to, I highly recommend doing this outside. It can be as simple as sitting on the patch of grass in front of your home or on a balcony where you can feel the fresh air. If that's not possible, try it sitting next to your houseplants.

THE PRACTICE

1. Sitting cross-legged on the ground, place your palms down on the ground next to you on each side.

2. As you breathe in through your nose, imagine raising earth energy from the ground as you bring your hands up around you and almost touch at the top.

3. Exhale through your mouth in an "O" shape, making a soft "phhh" sound, as you bring your palms down in front of your body and gently touch the ground in front of you.

4. Take your breaths slowly and intentionally. There is no rush.

5. Repeat seven times.

TIP

While you do this practice, you can visualize a golden ball of light around you. When you move your arms from the side of your body, you can envision that light surrounding your entire body. When you bring your hands down in front of your body, you can visualize a stream of light going in a straight line from the top of your head, down the center of your body, and then all the way down to the ground. This is you receiving earth energy, neutralizing it, and sending it back to the earth.

REFLECTION

🌿 How can you use this practice in your daily life?

🌿 What thoughts did you notice?

🌿 What sensations did you feel?

26   THE FULL BODY GROUNDING BREATH

Duration: A few seconds to 7 minutes

Call upon this technique anytime you'd like to:

- 🌱 Ground yourself
- 🌱 Recenter your energy
- 🌱 Connect to the Earth
- 🌱 Come back to your body
- 🌱 Relieve stress
- 🌱 Invite in relaxation
- 🌱 Calm your thoughts
- 🌱 Release nervousness

The Full Body Grounding Breath has the same philosophy as the Grounding Touch Breath, the previous technique, and essentially provides a very similar recalibration in the body. This time, we're adding in full body movement and connecting it all. Call upon this breath when you'd like to completely transmute your physical energy, cleanse your vibration, ground, and center yourself.

1. Stand comfortably upright with space to move your arms; place your arms by your sides.

2. Gently bend your knees while breathing in through your nose and imagine raising earth energy from the ground as you bring your hands up around you and almost touch at the top.

3. Exhale through your mouth in an "O" shape, making a soft "phhh" sound, as you bring your palms down across the front of your body while envisioning sending energy into the ground.

4. Repeat seven times.

TIP

You can use the same tip as the seated Grounding Touch Breath and this time, play around with drawing different colored balls of light around you.

REFLECTION

- How does this technique feel different standing up versus seated?

- What colors intuitively came to you?

- What sensations did you feel?

THE SMILING BREATH

Duration: A few seconds to 7 minutes

Call upon this technique anytime you'd like to:

- ⚘ Ground yourself
- ⚘ Feel joy
- ⚘ Recenter your energy
- ⚘ Cool the body
- ⚘ Relieve stress
- ⚘ Invite in relaxation
- ⚘ Calm your thoughts
- ⚘ Release nervousness

Smile! Did you know there is some serious science behind smiling? Yes! When you smile, powerful neurotransmitters get activated in your brain and send happiness chemicals throughout your body. Even when you're not actually feeling happy per se, putting a smile on your face can essentially trick your brain into believing that you are happy. When you feel it, you can be it!

Smiling releases endorphins, which are natural painkillers. These chemicals help the body relax and reduce physical pain. Your brain also releases neuropeptides, which are incredibly important for managing stress. Other chemicals like dopamine, serotonin, and oxytocin are also released, reducing the stress hormone cortisol. That sounds like we have a whole medicine cabinet at the ready just from putting on a smile, and I can get with that.

I'm not going to lie: when you first do this technique, you might feel very awkward! I know it's unnatural to smile like this and to hold your mouth this way. But trust that the signals in your body are being received. Your neurotransmitters are listening to you. And the oxygen that you're bringing in to distribute these feel-good hormones will make a world of difference after you finish this practice.

THE PRACTICE

1. Start wherever you are.
2. Smile with your upper and lower teeth gently touching each other.
3. Breathe in through your teeth for as long as it feels comfortable.
4. Breathe out through your teeth for as long as it feels comfortable.

TIPS

An awesome visual to use for this technique is yourself in front of the mirror! Trust me—you'll look very silly doing this, but as long as we're talking about smiling, laughing, being silly, and experiencing joy, you might as well get in front of the mirror and see what you look like.

Another great enhancement for this breathwork technique is to play some music that makes you smile. You're welcome to put on some jams, use headphones, or maybe even put on a comedy!

REFLECTION

- Did you notice any temperature changes in your body?

- What did you think of the sounds coming out of your mouth?

- What other sensations did you experience?

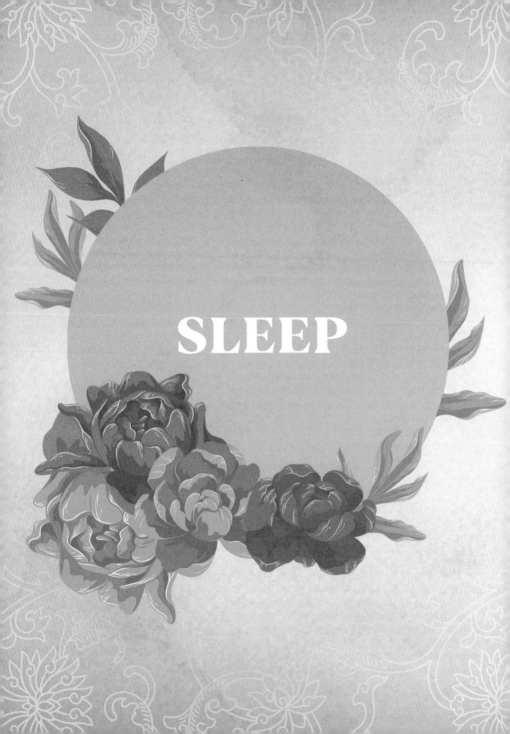

SLEEP

These powerful breathwork techniques promote rest and can improve the quality of your sleep. You might notice a change in your sleep patterns after keeping up with a consistent nighttime breathwork routine. Even if you still sleep the same number of hours, you'll notice a different quality in your sleep. Start to keep track of how you feel in the morning after you've been consistent with a nighttime breathwork routine.

I highly recommend setting yourself up to fall asleep after practicing these techniques! Do these techniques when you're all ready for bed and you won't have to get up to brush your teeth, put on your jammies, or turn off the lights.

If you do happen to fall asleep (likely!) after many of these practices, feel free to complete the reflection portion the following day.

Sleep tight.

THE 2-6-8 BREATH

Duration: 7 minutes

Call upon this technique anytime you'd like to:

🌱 Improve sleep

🌱 Invite calm

🌱 Feel peace and relaxation

🌱 Relieve stress and anxiety

I f you've had one of those chaotic days where you didn't get one second to yourself, this is the practice for you. You see, when we're really busy, our bodies move into go-go-go mode. We're problem solving, we're getting things done, we're on #bossmode, and all of that. But, if we're always in that mode, we can cause long-term harm to our bodies by overexerting ourselves. We're essentially not getting enough oxygen through our system to allow us to get optimal rest; instead, we're using up precious resources that can really tire us out in the long run.

The 2-6-8 Breath slows down the body, invites in calm, and improves sleep. This technique sends a signal to the body that you aren't in danger and can relax.

When you are ready to wind down for the night, set yourself up to rest, relax, and fall asleep with this technique. Having a comfy environment with blankets and pillows is great for this one.

THE PRACTICE

1. Sit or lie comfortably and close your eyes.
2. Breathe in through your mouth for two seconds as if you are gulping in air with a straw in two parts.
3. On your first breath, sip into your belly and feel your belly go all the way out.
4. Without exhaling, sip the second breath into your chest and feel your ribs expand. You can think in your mind "1, 2," as you take the two BIG sips of air.
5. Hold your breath for six seconds, counting down in your head: 6-5-4-3-2-1.
6. Exhale for eight seconds through your mouth with the same straw method, counting down in your head: 8-7-6-5-4-3-2-1.
7. Repeat for as long as you'd like.

TIP

A calming essential oil such as lavender is a great choice for this breathwork.

REFLECTION

🌿 How does your breath sound entering and leaving your vessel?

🌿 How can you practice surrendering your body?

🌿 Where can you release tension?

29

THE CANDLE BREATH FOR SLEEP

Duration: 2 to 7 minutes

**Call upon this
technique anytime
you'd like to:**

❀ Improve sleep

❀ Rest

❀ Relax

This is a similar exercise to the Candle Breath for Energy on page 97. You'll also be envisioning putting out a candle with your breath, but this time you'll be doing so as you welcome sleep, relaxation, total peace, and calm into your energetic body. This technique is perfect for curling up with a hot cup of tea and a good book, and right before calling it a night. Prepare your space—get your pillows, blankets, kitties, and puppies—and be prepared to be in bed for the rest of the night.

The Candle Breath for Sleep helps slow down your mind. If you're somebody who has a lot of thoughts right before going to bed, you can pair this breathing technique with some journaling right before bed or doing what's known as a brain dump. A brain dump helps you clear out all your thoughts onto a piece of paper so you can worry less and sleep better.

This gentle technique can also be done with an actual candle if you would like to. And in fact, many meditation and yoga practices include candles in breathwork and mindfulness meditation.

Just like in our previous candle technique, you'll be blowing your breath at a candle flame—either metaphorically or literally if you're using a real candle. But this time, your intention is not to put out the flame. You want to get as close to blowing out the flame without actually blowing out the flame. How can you balance the gentleness and the force of your breath to move and manipulate the flame without actually putting it out? If you're blowing too hard, you're going to put out the flame. If you're blowing too softly, then your air will not reach the flame. You want to figure out, metaphorically or literally, how hard you have to blow in order to gently make this flame dance. Now, it might be easier to use a real candle for this, and if so, be sure to put it out before going to sleep and be careful with fire.

THE PRACTICE

1. If you are using a real candle, sit up while you either hold or place the candle in a safe container in front of you. If you are using a metaphorical candle, feel free to sit or lie down.

2. Close your eyes if you aren't using a real candle; if you are using a real candle, keep your eyes open.

3. Breathe deeply in through your nose for five seconds and fill up your entire body with air.

4. Very gently, blow at the flame (imaginary or real) with your mouth without putting out the flame.

5. You can play around with the intensity, pace, and distance of your breath from the flame.

6. Repeat for as long as you like.

TIPS

If you're not using a candle for this practice, you can blow into your hands instead. Gently feel your breath touch your skin. Notice the temperature of your breath. Play around with blowing gently and also with a bit of force. You can move your hands closer or farther away from your mouth to see what feels good.

A white noise machine or a playlist with nature sounds is an incredible addition to this practice.

REFLECTION

❊ What did you notice about this (metaphorical or real) flame?

❊ What did you notice about your thoughts?

❊ What sensations did you experience after the practice?

30

THE EQUAL BREATH

Duration: 2 to 7 minutes

Call upon this technique anytime you'd like to:

- Improve sleep
- Rest
- Relax

To be honest, your body already does this right as you're about to go to sleep. It's not something that you truly need to learn how to do. But if you struggle with sleep, you may be holding your breath and not allowing yourself to fully go into that rest and relaxation mode that's needed for optimal sleep. Essentially, you can trick your body into believing that you are prepared for sleep even if you are not ready to go to bed.

The Equal Breath is exactly what it sounds like: you take equal breaths in and equal breaths out. You can do this technique through either your nose or your mouth. Most people prefer to do this through the nose because it feels more natural, and it helps to not dry out the mouth, especially if you are comfy in bed. This breathwork also produces sounds. Really embrace and enjoy the soothing sounds that your body naturally makes and lean in to how relaxing and comforting that can feel.

THE PRACTICE

1. Lie down and slowly close your eyes.
2. Take a breath for five seconds through your nose or mouth directed toward your throat.
3. Exhale through your nose or mouth for five seconds and feel your body empty out.
4. Repeat for as long as you like.

TIPS

You can place a calming essential oil, such as lavender or rose, on the palms of your hands and rub them together. As you're practicing and falling asleep, keep your hands somewhere on your body that feels right, perhaps on your belly, or one hand on your belly and one on your heart.

A white noise machine or a playlist with nature sounds is a great accompaniment to this breathwork.

REFLECTION

- How different does it feel breathing from your nose versus your mouth?
- Are you rushing on either the inhale or the exhale? Try to inhale and exhale at the same pace.
- How long were you able to practice?

THE OCEAN BREATH

Duration: 2 to 7 minutes

Call upon this technique anytime you'd like to:

❁ Improve sleep

❁ Rest

❁ Relax

❁ Cool the body

The Ocean Breath, or Ujjayi Pranayama in Sanskrit, is another popular relaxation breathing technique in yoga. This is known as the Ocean Breath because it resembles the sound of ocean waves rolling back and forth · onto shore. This peaceful, gentle sound brings a cooling effect and releases tension, calms the nerves, and regulates body temperature.

In yoga, this is part of a breathwork technique that helps connect the movements, philosophy, and breath of yoga. Many people use this technique at the end of their practice because it helps bring the body back to center, cleanses the mind, and really brings a sensation of peace to every single cell. In this technique, we breathe into our skull rather than breathing from the nose with strong inhales. You'll feel the air going down the back of your throat and then into your chest and belly, in that order.

You'll also sense a cooling sensation in the body. This can be really powerful right before sleep because if you've been very active or busy during the day, there is a lot of energy that has moved through you. This cooling effect helps you relax and release muscle tension. The Ocean Breath is also great for activating the parasympathetic nervous system, which is a perfect coupling for going to sleep. This technique helps you get deeper sleep and a better quality of sleep throughout the night. You might also notice differences in your dreams when practicing this type of breathing.

When you first start doing this breath, you might feel a resistance to breathing into your throat. It might feel like your throat is itching. That's okay. You'll get used to the sensation as you continue with the practice. It's important to breathe into the throat instead of directly into your brain, because you're not trying to awaken your brain right now; you're asking your brain to rest and relax so that you can chill and go to sleep. While you let your brain relax, it'll help you transition from a beta (active) state to an alpha (sleepy) state, and eventually into a deep theta (restorative, meditative) state. By the time you get there, your body will naturally take over the breathing and you won't have to think about this technique while you fall into deep, peaceful sleep.

THE PRACTICE

1. Lie down and gently close your eyes. Get as comfortable as possible.
2. To begin, take a few breaths that feel natural to you.
3. Take a long inhale in through your nose into your throat, filling up your body as much as possible.
4. Slowly exhale out of your mouth while making a near silent "ha" sound.
5. Continue this pattern until your body naturally returns to your regular breathing or you fall asleep.

TIP

Ocean Breath often creates a cooling sensation in the body as it promotes sleep. Use blankets over you or wear comfortable clothes that cover you before you begin.

REFLECTION

✤ What sounds did you notice?

✤ Did you notice any shifts in temperature?

✤ What sensations did you feel?

THE LULLABY BREATH

32

Duration: 2 to 7 minutes

Call upon this technique anytime you'd like to:

✤ Improve sleep

✤ Rest

✤ Relax

The Lullaby Breath combines all the features and benefits of the Humming Breath (see page 124) and makes it easy to use for sleep. In the same way that being sung to sleep is comforting and relaxing, the sound of your own voice and breath carries the same sentiment. It's pretty hard to sing yourself to sleep; you might try it, but it might keep you up even longer!

Humming is a gentle, soothing sensation that helps calm and relax and gently, vibrationally cradles you in your own sonic comfort. If you're used to hearing snoring, this may not feel too relaxing for you right off the bat, but the self-soothing technique can be a powerful way to gently lull yourself to sleep.

THE PRACTICE

1. Lie down and close your eyes, making sure you are comfortable.
2. Take a natural breath in through your nose.
3. With your mouth closed, hum as you exhale fully, taking as long as you want.
4. Repeat as many times as you'd like.

TIP

Play around with humming sounds that bring comfort to you.

REFLECTION

- How did the humming feel?
- Did you notice a shift in your voice?
- What did you notice about your thoughts?

33

THE COUNTING BREATH

Duration: 2 to 7 minutes

Call upon this technique anytime you'd like to:

- 🌿 Improve sleep
- 🌿 Rest
- 🌿 Relax

This breathwork technique is meant to help you keep it as natural as possible right before going to bed. Just as we started this guide with a simple natural breathing technique, we'll wrap up the same way. For this breathwork, you choose the length of your inhales and exhales. You get to choose the experience you want. The point of this breathing method is to help your body naturally recalibrate and help you mindfully, intuitively, and intentionally bring the precious gift of breath back into your body.

THE PRACTICE

1. Lie down and close your eyes.

2. To begin, take a few breaths that feel natural to you.

3. Take in a long inhale through your nose, counting from one in your mind until you are done taking in this natural inhale.

4. Exhale out through your nose, counting from one in your mind until you are done exhaling.

5. Repeat as long as you'd like.

TIP

There is no right or wrong length to your inhales or exhales. Tune in to your body's natural rhythm as you breathe in and breathe out.

REFLECTION

❀ How did the natural pace of your breath feel?

❀ Was there a difference between your inhales and exhales?

❀ What thoughts floated through?

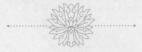

Breathwork Tool Kit

There you have it: thirty-three incredibly easy yet potent breathwork techniques you're going to be showing off around the neighborhood. But really, please show them around the neighborhood because we can all use access to how good these are!

Let's create a Breathwork Tool Kit, which will help you pick and choose your favorite and most useful practices as they relate to your life. Use the questions in this section to reflect on your breathing journey. Write down your answers in your personal journal or on a separate piece of paper.

- What differences did you feel in your breathing?

- Are there any changes in the way your body takes in the breath?

- What have you noticed about yourself in your everyday life as you've implemented breathwork?

- Which techniques were your favorites?

- When will you use these techniques in your own life?

- Which couple of practices can you commit to learning very well so that you can show them to others?

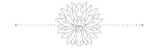

Further Resources/Extras

Woohoo! You've learned so many amazing breathwork techniques and are practicing mindful breathing! Big congratulations to you for keeping up a consistent practice, trying out different techniques, and staying with it going forward. I'd love to see you practicing these techniques.

Share your practice with me and stay in touch on Instagram @shanila.sattar and tag #breathworkguide when you share your breathing techniques with your community.

Go to www.alwaysplay.org/breathe for videos to practice the exercises I've marked throughout the book with 🪷, see the breathwork demonstrated, get more information, learn about breathwork facilitation, or continue your practice with me.

Happy breathing!

Acknowledgments

I'd love to thank all my breathwork facilitator students, mentees, and those who have come to breathe with me over the years for keeping me a continuous student and for informing this body of work. You've inspired me to express breathwork practically so that all of our family, friends, and communities can actually use these wonderful practices in daily life.

Thank you to my own family, baby Kebabu, bestie Gogo, Annie, Spencer, and all my houseplants for giving me life and support in birthing this breathwork guide. Thank you to my Boro Nanu for always inspiring me from far away with grace, elegance, and curiosity.

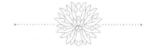

About the Author

Shanila Sattar is the founder of AlwaysPlay Studios, where she trains breathwork facilitators and sound healers, and mentors aspiring healers through her Integrative Healing Academy and Healing Arts Practitioner Program. She is a women's researcher and the creator of FLOW Breathwork, a somatic practice that uses the breath with movement and dance. She thrives in supporting the healing arts and in expanding accessible holistic wellness tools like breathwork and sound healing. Shanila hosts a top-rated show called *The Playground Podcast,* which is all about spiritual exploration, self-healing, personal development, and intuitive entrepreneurship.

Connect and practice breathwork with Shanila on her YouTube channel and Instagram @shanila.sattar. Come learn more about breathwork at www.alwaysplay.org.

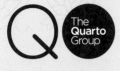

Inspiring | Educating | Creating | Entertaining

Brimming with creative inspiration, how-to projects, and useful information to enrich your everyday life, quarto.com is a favorite destination for those pursuing their interests and passions.

First published in 2022 by Rock Point, an imprint of The Quarto Group,
142 West 36th Street, 4th Floor, New York, NY 10018, USA
T (212) 779-4972 F (212) 779-6058 www.Quarto.com

Rock Point titles are also available at discount for retail, wholesale, promotional, and bulk purchase. For details, contact the Special Sales Manager by email at specialsales@quarto.com or by mail at The Quarto Group, Attn: Special Sales Manager, 100 Cummings Center Suite 265D, Beverly, MA 01915 USA.

10 9 8 7 6 5 4

ISBN: 978-1-63106-827-0

Library of Congress Cataloging-in-Publication Data

Names: Sattar, Shanila, author.
Title: Breathe : 33 simple breathwork practices / Shanila Sattar.
Description: New York, NY : Rock Point, 2022. | Series: Mind body soul |
    Summary: "Breathe will teach you how targeted breathwork affects the body and mind
    and how to make the most of it with simple, hassle-free exercises"-- Provided by publisher.
Identifiers: LCCN 2021042357 (print) | LCCN 2021042358 (ebook) | ISBN
    9781631068270 (hardcover) | ISBN 9780760373729 (ebook)
Subjects: LCSH: Mind and body. | Breathing exercises. | Self-help techniques.
Classification: LCC BF161 .S228 2022 (print) | LCC BF161 (ebook) | DDC 613/.192--dc23/eng/20211007
LC record available at https://lccn.loc.gov/2021042357
LC ebook record available at https://lccn.loc.gov/2021042358

Publisher: Rage Kindelsperger
Creative Director: Laura Drew
Managing Editor: Cara Donaldson
Editor: Keyla Pizarro-Hernández
Cover and Interior Design: Amelia LeBarron

Printed in China

This book provides general information on the breath and breathwork techniques. However, it should not be relied upon as recommending or promoting any specific diagnosis or method of treatment for a particular condition, and it is not intended as a substitute for medical advice or for direct diagnosis and treatment of a medical condition by a qualified physician. Readers who have questions about a particular condition, possible treatments for that condition, or possible reactions from the condition or its treatment should consult a physician or other qualified healthcare professional.